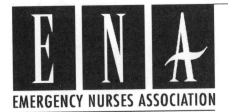

EMERGENCY NURSES ASSOCIATION

ADVANCED · PRACTICE · NURSING

Current Practice Issues in Emergency Care

Second Edition

KENDALL/HUNT PUBLISHING COMPANY
4050 Westmark Drive Dubuque, Iowa 52002

Disclaimer

The authors, editors, and publisher have checked with reliable resources in regards to providing information that is complete and accurate. Due to the continual evolution of knowledge, treatment modalities, and drug therapies, ENA cannot warranty that the information, in every aspect, is current. ENA is not responsible for any errors, omissions, or for the results obtained, from use of such information. Please check with your health care institution regarding policies and practices relating to medications and nursing practice.

CONTENTS

ACKNOWLEDGMENTS

Editor

Vicki A. Keough, RN-CS, PhD, ACNP, CCRN
Associate Professor
Loyola University Chicago
Niehoff School of Nursing
Maywood, IL

Contributing Authors

Marlene Angelico, RN, MSN, ANP
Nurse Practitioner, Emergency Department
Evanston Northwestern Healthcare
Evanston, IL

Susan A. Barnason, PhD, RN, CEN, CCRN,
    APRN, BC
Associate Professor
University of Nebraska Medical Center:
    College of Nursing
Lincoln, NE

Susan M. Bednar, RN, MSN, ANP
Manager-Fast Track Services
Evanston Northwestern Healthcare
Evanston, IL

Barbara W. Bollenberg, RN, PhD(c), CEN
Staff Nurse, Emergency Department
Edward Hines Veterans Administration Hospital
Hines, IL

Frank L. Cole, PhD, RN, CEN, CS, FNP, FAAN,
    FAANP
Professor of Nursing, Division Head
    of Emergency Care and
Director, Emergency Nurse Practitioner
    Education
The University of Texas Health Science
    at Houston
Houston, TX

Darcy Egging, RN, MS, CS-ANP, CEN
Nurse Practitioner
Valley Emergency Care, Inc.
Delnor-Community Hospital
Geneva, IL

Mary E. Hardesty, RN, MS, FNP
Director of Education
Emergency Nurse Practitioner
Evanston Northwestern Healthcare
Evanston, IL

Karen Sue Hoyt, RN, MN, PhD(c), CEN
Masters Entry Program in Nursing Coordinator
Assistant Clinical Professor
Hahn School of Nursing and Health Science
University of San Diego
San Diego, CA

Judith A. Jennrich, RN-CS, PhD, ACNP, CCRN
Associate Professor
Loyola University Chicago
Niehoff School of Nursing
Maywood, IL

Vicki A. Keough, RN-CS, PhD, ACNP, CCRN
Associate Professor
Loyola University Chicago
Niehoff School of Nursing
Maywood, IL

Gail Pisarcik Lenehan, RN, EdD, FAAN
Editor, *Journal of Emergency Nursing*
Hingham, MA

Jean A. Proehl, RN, MN, CEN, CCRN
Emergency Clinical Nurse Specialist
Dartmouth-Hitchcock Medical Center
Lebanon, NH

Elda G. Ramirez, MSN, RN, FNP, CS, CEN
Assistant Professor, Clinical Nursing
University of Texas School of Nursing
Houston, TX

Doris A. Rasmussen, MSN, RN, CCRN, CEN, CS, CCNS
Clinical Nurse Specialist
Bryan LGH Medical Center
Lincoln, NE

Suzanne Rita, RN, MSN
Lecturer
Old Dominion University School of Nursing
Norfolk, VA

Janice S. Rogers, MS, RN, CS, PNP
Pediatric Nurse Practitioner
Pediatric Emergency Department
Golisano Children's Hospital at Strong
Assistant Professor of Nursing
University of Rochester
Rochester, NY

Lynn Scarbrough, RN, MSN, ACNP
Emergency Nurse Practitioner
Emergency Care Group, Inc.
Lake Zurich, IL

Edwin W. Schaefer, ND, RN, FNP
Emergency Nurse Practitioner
Delnor-Community Hospital
Geneva, IL

Sharon Schultz, RN, BS, MPH, CCPSI
Director, Nursing Administration
RUSH-Copley Medical Center
Aurora, IL

T. Smith, RN, MS, CS, FNP-C
Family Nurse Practitioner
Naperville, IL

Rebecca A. Steinmann, RN, MS, CEN, CCRN, CCNS
Clinical Educator, Emergency Department
Children's Memorial Hospital
Chicago, IL

Elisabeth K. Weber, RN, MA, CEN, CCNS
Administrative Coordinator, Children's Memorial Hospital
Independent Consultant in Emergency Services
Chicago, IL

Barbara A. Weintraub, RN, MSN, MPH, PCCNP, CEN
Coordinator, Pediatric Emergency Services
Northwest Community Hospital
Arlington Heights, IL

Kathleen Evanovich Zavotsky, MS, RN, CCRN, CNS, C, CEN
Clinical Nurse Specialist, Emergency Department
Robert Wood Johnson University Hospital
New Brunswick, NJ

Reviewers

Chris M. Gisness, RN, MSN, CEN, CS, FNP-C
Associate Provider
Department of Emergency Medicine
Emory University
Atlanta, GA

Suzanne M. Wall, RN, MS, CEN, FNP
Nurse Practitioner
Sentara Williamsburg Community Hospital
Occupational Health Center
Orlando, FL

Mary Ellen Wilson, RN, MS, CEN, FNP
Clinical Education Specialist, Emergency Services
New Hanover Health Network
Wilmington, NC

Staff Liaison

Donna Massey, RN, MSN, CCNS
Director, Educational Services
Emergency Nurses Association
Des Plaines, IL

A special thanks to the following individuals who made the first edition of the Advanced Nursing Practice manual possible.

Connie Dishon, RN, MAN, CEN

Darcy Egging, RN, MS, ANP, CEN, MICN

Linda L. Larson, RN, PhD, FNP, CEN

Suzanne Rita, RN, MAN, CEN, CNS

Ellen Ruja, RN, MAN, CEN

Sheila Sanning Shea, RN, MSN, ANP, CEN

T. Smith, RN, MS, CEN

Patricia A. Southard, RN, MN, JD

Rebecca A. Steinmann, RN, MS, CEN, CCRN

Nancy Stonis, RN, BSN, MJ, CEN

Paula Tanabe, RN, PhD(c), CEN, CCRN

Suzanne M. Wall, MS, RNC, CEN

PART ONE

INTRODUCTION

1

ADVANCED PRACTICE NURSING: A HISTORICAL PERSPECTIVE

Janice S. Rogers, MS, RN, CS, PNP

Although there is evidence of persons who provided care and comfort for sick people in prehistoric times, Florence Nightingale is credited with beginning nursing as a specific professional entity. Her efforts and persistence in the mid-1800s formalized and promoted the nursing role. Subsequent nursing development was often slow, and prolonged setbacks occurred. Nightingale's recommendation that nursing education be provided through professional institutions that were not associated with hospitals did not come to fruition until the late 1900s.[1] Nursing did eventually advance, however, not only as a professional entity in itself, but also in extended settings, duties, and roles.

Specific advanced nursing practice specialties were developed in the mid- to late-1800s. Nurse specialists earned their rank through completion of a postgraduate course in a specialty area or clinical experience and expertise.[2] Nurse anesthesia, the oldest advanced nursing specialty, dates back to the mid-1800s, the beginning of anesthesia itself.[3] Nurses as midwives increased in the 1920s with the development of community-based maternity centers in New York City and the Frontier Nursing Service in the economically depressed Appalachian mountain area.[3–5] Other nursing specialty areas included tuberculosis, operating room, communicable diseases, and dietetics. Nurses also expanded their role to include specific tasks. For example, in the 1930s and 1940s, experienced nurse technical specialists were specially trained to perform x-rays and laboratory tests.[6] These specialties provided the framework for the proliferation and development of later advanced nursing practice roles.

Clinical Nurse Specialists

The clinical nurse specialist (CNS) role was formalized in the 1940s. Although there was disagreement about the specific origin of the concept, most parties agreed that the CNS or "nurse clinician" title described a nurse with advanced clinical competence and education at the master's level.[7–10] The CNS role focused on improving the quality of care delivered to patients, primarily in institutional settings, and on keeping the expert nurse at the bedside. Specialties were subsequently developed in response to the following societal forces: (1) an increase in specialty-related information and technological advances, and (2) the public's needs and interests of the times.[8]

CNS role development was hampered by the lack of bacheloriate-prepared nurses who were eligible for postgraduate education and by the limited availability of CNS programs. The first CNS master's program was not established until 1954 at Rutgers University.[3] Because of the paucity of educational programs, a multitude of nurses claimed the specialist title without appropriate academic credentials. This, in addition to the variety of specialties and individual roles, fostered role confusion surrounding the CNS position.

Over the next several decades, the CNS role flourished with relative ease. Because the role developed within the domain of nursing itself, there were few turf wars with other professions. The role was also strongly supported by nursing leaders and educators. The inclusion of CNS students in the Professional Nurse Traineeship Program in 1963 and the Nurse Training Act (Title VIII of the Public Health Service Act) of 1965 fostered clinical nursing specialization through financial support of graduate-level clinical specialist education. The positive effect of the CNS role on nursing care improvements and patient outcomes was validated by a variety of research studies.[11-16]

Certification of registered nurses (RNs) and CNSs by the American Nurses Association (ANA) began in the mid-1970s. However, many of the specialty certification exams were at the basic level. Advanced practice nursing certifications became available much later for many, but not all, specialties. Neither basic nor advanced certification is available for some specialties.[3]

The onset of health care cost containment in the mid-1980s challenged CNSs to prove their worth financially. Because there was no direct billing or reimbursement for CNS care, their salaries were built into general nursing or hospital budgets. It was difficult to validate direct cost savings of clinical specialists involved in nursing orientation and education, role modeling excellent care, and patient education. Numerous CNS positions were eliminated because their cost effectiveness could not be proved. By the mid-1990s the demand for and number of graduate CNS programs had sharply declined,[17] not only in response to cost containment but also because of the proliferation of nurse practitioner (NP) programs and positions and the growing emphasis on primary care. Many CNS roles were reengineered to serve the social and political needs of the times as well as the needs of patients.[18-19] The flexibility of the CNS role facilitated its survival and effectiveness. In 1998, the National Advisory Council on Nurse Education and Practice stated, "The CNS provider is a viable member of the evolving health care delivery team, even as the direct and indirect roles of the CNS continue to change, adapting to changing population needs and the health care market place."[20]

The blending of the CNS and the NP roles has been a topic of much discussion over the past 20 years. In 1986, the ANA Council of CNSs (CCNS) and the Council of Primary Health Care NPs (CPHCNP) met to discuss the commonalities between the two roles.[21] The two councils merged in 1991 to form the Council of Nurses in Advanced Practice (CNAP). The CNAP addressed the collective needs of all advanced practice nurses (APNs). Subsequently, the ANA and the National League for Nursing recom-

mended the blending of the CNS and NP roles by the year 2010. Advantages of a blended role primarily include cost effectiveness, both in educational and health care settings, and a more defined role for nursing in current health reform.[22-25] One role or title would foster political influence and public acceptance of APNs,[19] increase the independence of APNs,[26] and facilitate third-party reimbursement and broader prescriptive privileges for CNSs.[23,25,27,28] Disadvantages of a blended role include the deleterious effect of title change on the advances already made by NPs in reimbursement, credentialing, and public and governmental awareness; the potential loss of many positive CNS roles, particularly in program development, education, and support of nurses at the bedside; and the role strain and confusion of combining two roles by one individual.[22,29] The controversy about the effects of a blended role on quality of care, the advancement of nursing, and the current health care system continues today.

CNS functions in the emergency department (ED) have traditionally included expert nursing care, orientation, in-service, continuing education, and program planning and development. Clinical specialists in primary or acute care of adults, psychiatric or mental health, pediatrics, and trauma have successfully performed these functions in the ED. Although administrators generally supported the CNS role, resistance did occur. Threatened head nurses or staff nurses often challenged the expertise of CNSs, who did not routinely prove their abilities at the bedside. A greater threat to the CNS role occurred during the tight financial times of the 1990s. Many CNS positions were lost to cost-cutting measures or restructured to nurse practitioner roles. The work of the CNS was often relegated to experienced staff nurses or nurse managers. Because staff nurses' time was primarily spent with patient care, educational efforts and program planning suffered. Despite the obstacles, many CNSs have survived in EDs that value and financially support the traditional role. Other CNSs have redesigned their roles as case managers, expert direct nursing caregivers for discreet populations, or coordinators of programs serving specific complex or high-risk populations, such as patients with suspected myocardial infarctions.

Nurse Practitioners

The birth of the nurse practitioner role in 1965 is credited to Loretta Ford, RN, Ed.D., and Henry Silver, MD, at the University of Colorado. Their demonstration project responded to the social climate of the 1960s: (1) health manpower shortages, especially in pediatrics and family care; (2) maldistribution of resources leading to a lack of primary care in high-risk urban and rural settings; (3) rising health care costs; (4) projected increases in health care demand due to the passage of Medicare and Medicaid; and (5) the quest for nursing autonomy and accountability in the care of both sick and well people.[30–34] The first NPs were trained during a 4-month, intensive postbaccalaureate educational and practical training period to provide comprehensive well-child care and to manage minor health care problems. Although this training expanded the role of the nurse beyond the boundaries of traditional nursing, basic nursing tenets of health maintenance, wellness, and prevention were retained. The pediatric nurse practitioner (PNP) was *not* intended to substitute for the physician. Dr. Ford envisioned a collaborative and collegial role between the physician and PNP.[32–33] An evaluative study indicated that the newly trained PNPs were highly competent in the assessment and management of most of the children seen, and their use increased the number of children served in private practices by 33%.[3,33]

The nurse practitioner movement rapidly spread to other specialties and to other settings, including the acute care arena. In 1969, a 4-month family NP program (Primex) was developed at the University of Washington.[35] Neonatal ICU and cardiothoracic surgery NPs appeared in the 1970s. Although nurse practitioners filled many gaps in health care, the utilization of NPs varied by institution and by region of the country. In areas of high demand, NPs were recruited from unit staff or were transferred from ambulatory care. The requirements for entry into practice and the educational preparation of NPs were highly variable.

NP programs quickly developed in emergency care. Mildred Fincke, Virginia Musick, and Barbara Cline initiated the Emergency/Ambulatory Nurse Practitioner Program in 1972 at the Allegheny General Hospital in Pittsburgh, Pennsylvania. Participants in this program were trained to assume many of the routine tasks and responsibilities of physicians, but were not allowed to make medical diagnoses or prescribe medications.[36] In 1975, Linda Larson and her team advanced the role further by designing an independent emergency department nurse practitioner (EDNP) program.[37] Nurses who completed their intensive 6-month educational program went on to provide independent emergency care in hospital-based freestanding emergency care centers in Colorado. These centers successfully operated for 8 years, when physicians took over the care. The more costly physician-run centers lost favor with the public and subsequently closed. Other programs developed in the 1970s utilized NPs in triage and walk-in clinics or fast-track settings.[38–40] Throughout the first two decades of NP care, there was great variability in the utilization of emergency NPs, educational preparation, and the degree of NP autonomy.

Acceptance of the NP role did not occur easily. With the encroachment of NP practice into the medical field, many physicians and residents doubted the NPs' abilities and strongly resisted their utilization. Even nurses challenged the new NPs, accusing them of abandoning nursing. Loretta Ford was disheartened by the resistance of her academic colleagues. Rather than usurping the physician role, Ford viewed the PNP program as reclaiming the original public health nurses' independent role in well-child care that was lost in the 1930s when the American Academy of Pediatrics claimed well-child care as their domain.[41] Although early research data justified the efficacy of the NP role in comparison to physicians,[42–45] the debate about NP practice continued. In 1986 the Office of Technology Assessment eliminated much of the dissension with respect to primary care NPs. After a comprehensive review of the literature, they concluded that primary and ambulatory care NPs "within their areas of competence . . . provide care whose quality is equivalent to that of care provided by physicians" and are "more adept than physicians at providing services that depend on communication with patients and preventive action."[42] Despite this pronouncement and the positive research data, acceptance of NPs is still a concern today, especially in acute and critical care areas.

Multiple barriers to NP care persisted, causing some to fear for the survival of the NP role. These obstacles included role confusion; multiple entry levels to practice; variable educational programs; lack of consensus on name and titling; limited consumer awareness; lack of energy to organize, unite, and advance the NP role; legal and legislative ambiguities; financial constraints; threatened surplus of MDs; and territorial issues between MDs and NPs.[46] However, NPs rose to the challenge, and the role has survived, despite these roadblocks. Progress has been slow, but important changes have occurred. In the late 1970s, the ANA declared the baccalaureate to be the appropriate level of education for entry into basic nursing practice,[47] and the National League for Nursing supported advanced education for NPs.[48] In 1984, the ANA passed a resolution requiring graduate preparation for entry into advanced nursing practice by 1990.[49] Nurse practitioners organized to promote legislative changes, set standards, define NP credentialing issues, and gain visibility. Despite the initial financial successes of NP programs, their cost effectiveness deteriorated because NPs were forced into more dependence on physicians to obtain reimbursement for services.[31,50,51] This presented another obstacle to overcome. Interestingly, many physicians were highly supportive of NPs' quest for third-party reimbursement to improve access to care and to provide the complementary services of NPs, such as health counseling, maintenance, and prevention. Although some issues have been resolved, many remain. The work continues to utilize NP strengths to their fullest capacity.

Where Do We Go from Here?

It is very interesting to look back at history only to find that many of the problems that fostered the growth of advanced practice nursing in years past are the same as today's dilemmas. The cost of care is rising at rapid rates. There is still a shortage and maldistribution of health care manpower. The urban poor and the rural populations are still underserved. Numerous patients are under- or uninsured. Specialists are abundant, whereas primary care providers are still in short supply. The

size of resident programs is decreasing, and resident hours are being curtailed. Despite the prevalence of managed care, the numbers of patient visits to EDs are rising. Poor access to care continues to inflate nonurgent visits to the ED. Overcrowded EDs and prolonged waiting times continue to frustrate the public. Many patient populations are not well served by the emergency system (or nonsystem) of care. Interrelationships between the ED and prehospital care, specialty services, primary care providers, and the public are often difficult at best. The explosion of new technology persists. Overwhelming? Yes! But APNs continue to seek new solutions to the challenges of health care because of their commitment to provide the best service possible for emergency patients.

How can APNs proceed in this chaotic environment? First, ED APNs need to know their history and their current state of affairs. A summary of APN history has been presented in this chapter. The remainder of the manual discusses APNs' present status and current issues. Second, APNs need to capitalize on the multiple opportunities available to advance nursing practice and improve the care of ED patients. Chaos is opportunity! And ED nurses, by their nature, thrive on chaos! APNs have proven their worth as providers, as change agents, as educators, and as researchers. APNs need to identify the gaps in their health care settings and develop programs accordingly. There may be a need for an NP-operated fast track, additional coverage of acutely ill or trauma patients, a follow-up program for ED patients, a telemedicine program for outlying areas, Web-based education for busy staff nurses, or an injury prevention program. The ideas are endless! Third, APNs need to foster legislation that allows them to use their talents in emergency care in a cost-effective way. This manual provides a wealth of knowledge about the APN role in emergency care. But it is up to individual APNs to step up to the plate and utilize this knowledge to provide the best care possible for emergency patients!

REFERENCES

1. Doheny, M. O., Cook, C. B., & Stopper, M. C. (1997). *The discipline of nursing: An introduction* (4th ed.). Stamford, CT: Appleton & Lange.

2. Dewitt, K. (1900). Specialties in nursing. *American Journal of Nursing, 1*, 14–17.

3. Bigbee, J. L., & Amidi-Nouri, A. (2000). History and evolution of advanced practice nursing practice. In A. B. Hamric, J. A. Spross, & C. M. Hanson (Eds.), *Advanced nursing practice: An integrative approach* (2nd ed., pp. 3–32). Philadelphia: Saunders.

4. Breckenridge, M. (1952). *Wide neighborhoods: A study of the frontier nursing service.* New York: Harper.

5. Varney, H. (1987). *Nurse midwifery* (2nd ed.). Boston: Blackwell Scientific.

6. Anesthesia? X-ray? Laboratory? (1941). *American Journal of Nursing, 41*(5), 567–568.

7. Norris, D. M. (1977). One perspective on the nurse practitioner movement. In A. Jacox & C. Norris (Eds.), *Organizing for independent nursing practice* (pp. 21–33). New York: Appleton-Century-Crofts.

8. Peplau, H. E. (1965). Specialization in professional nursing. *Nursing Science, 3,* 268–287.

9. Reiter, F. (1966). The nurse clinician. *American Journal of Nursing, 66,* 274–280.

10. Smoyak, S. A. (1976). Specialization in nursing: From then to now. *Nursing Outlook, 24,* 676–681.

11. Ayers, R. (1971). Effects and development of the role of the clinical nurse specialist. In R. Ayers (Ed.), *The clinical nurse specialist: An experiment in role effectiveness and role development* (pp. 32–49). Duarte, CA: City of Hope National Medical Center.

12. Georgopoulos, B. S., & Christman, L. (1970). The clinical nurse specialist: A role model. *American Journal of Nursing, 70,* 1030–1039.

13. Georgopoulos, B. S., & Jackson, M. M. (1970). Nursing kardex behavior in an experimental study of patient units with and without specialists. *Nursing Research, 19,* 196–218.

14. Georgopoulos, B. S., & Sana, M. (1971). Clinical nurse specialization and intershift report behavior. *American Journal of Nursing, 71,* 538–545.

15. Girouard, S. (1978). The role of the clinical nurse specialist as change agent: An experiment in preoperative teaching. *International Journal of Nursing Studies, 15,* 57–65.

16. Little, D. E., & Carnevali, D. (1967). Nurse specialist effect on tuberculosis. *Nursing Research, 16,* 321–326.

17. American Association of Colleges in Nursing. (1999). *Enrollment and graduations in baccalaureate and graduate programs in nursing.* Washington, DC: Author.

18. Quaal, S. J. (1999). Clinical nurse specialist: Role restructuring to advanced practice registered nurse. *Critical Care Nursing Quarterly, 21,* 37–49.

19. Schroer, D. (1991). Case management: Clinical nurse specialist and nurse practitioner, converging roles. *Clinical Nurse Specialist, 5*(4), 89–94.

20. National Advisory Council on Nurse Education and Practice. (1998). *Report to the Secretary of Health and Human Services: Federal support for the preparation of the clinical nurse specialist workforce through Title VIII.* Washington, DC: U.S. Department of Health and Human Services.

21. Redding, B. A. (1994, Spring/Summer). Titling and the advanced practice nurse. *Advanced practice nurse,* 7–8.

22. Page, N. E., & Arena, D. M. (1994). Rethinking the merger of the clinical nurse specialist and the nurse practitioner roles. *Image: Journal of nursing scholarship, 26*(4), 315–318.

23. Kitzman, H. (1989). The CNS and the nurse practitioner. In A. B. Hamric & J. A. Spross (Eds.), *The clinical nurse specialist in theory and practice* (pp. 379–394). Philadelphia: Saunders.

24. Mallison, M. (1993). Nurses as house staff. *American Journal of Nursing, 93,* 7.

25. Sawyers, J. E. (1993). Defining your role in ambulatory care: Clinical nurse specialist or nurse practitioner. *Clinical Nurse Specialist, 7*(1), 4–7.

26. Hunsberger, M., Mitchell, A., Blatz, S., Paes, B., Pinelli, J., Southwell, D., et al. (1992). Definition of an advanced nursing practice role in the NICU: The clinical nurse specialist/neonatal practitioner. *Clinical Nurse Specialist, 6*(2), 91–96.

27. Elder, R. G., & Bullough, B. (1990). Nurse practitioners and clinical nurse specialists: Are the roles merging? *Clinical Nurse Specialist, 4*(2), 78–84.

28. Forbes, K. E., Rafson, J., Spross, J. A., & Kozlowski, D. (1990). The clinical nurse specialist and nurse practitioner: Core curriculum survey results. *Clinical Nurse Specialist, 4*(2), 63–66.

29. Pearson, L. J., & Stallmeyer, J. (1987). Opposition to title change overwhelming. *Nurse Practitioner, 12*(5), 10, 15.

30. Brown, E. L. (1971). *Nursing reconsidered: A study of change: Vol. 2. The professional role in community nursing.* Philadelphia: Lippincott.

31. Edwards, C. C. (1974). A candid look at health manpower problems. *Journal of Medical Education, 49*(1), 19–26.

32. Ford, L. C. (1997). Advanced practice nursing: A deviant comes of age. *Heart and Lung, 26*(2), 87–91.

33. Ford, L. C., & Silver, H. K. (1967). The expanded role of the nurse in child care. *Nursing Outlook, 15,* 43–45.

34. Lee, P. R. (1966). New demands for medical manpower. *JAMA, 198*(10), 165–167.

35. Walker, A. E. (1972). PRIMEX—the family nurse practitioner program. *Nursing Outlook, 20*(1), 28–31.

36. Fincke, M. K. (1975). A new dimension in emergency nursing. *Journal of Emergency Nursing, 1*(5), 45–52.

37. Barnett, S. E., & Larson, L. (1975). Rural practitioners: A new community student health program. *Rocky Mountain Medical Journal, 75*(3), 151–155.

38. Buchanan, L., & Powers, R. D. (1997). Establishing an NP-staffed minor emergency area. *The Nurse Practitioner, 22*(4), 175–187.

39. Roglieri, J. L. (1975). Multiple expanded roles for nurses in urban emergency rooms. *Archives of Internal Medicine, 135,* 1401–1404.

40. Winston, S. (1981). Nurse practitioners in the emergency department: A case study of the Washington Hospital Center. *Hospital Topics, 59*(4), 10–13.

41. Ford, L. C. (1991). Advanced nursing practice: Future of the nurse practitioner. In L. H. Aiken & C. M. Fagin (Eds.), *Charting nursing's future: Agenda for the 1990s* (pp. 287–299). New York: Lippincott.

42. Congress of the United States, Office of Technology Assessment. (1986). *Nurse practitioners, physician assistants, and certified nurse-midwives: A policy analysis* (Health Technology case study 37, OTA-HCS-37). Washington, DC: U.S. Government Printing Office.

43. Edmonds, M. W. (1978). Evaluation of nurse practitioner effectiveness and overview of the literature. *Evaluation and the Health Professions, 1*(1), 69–82.

44. Feldman, M. J., Ventura, M. R., & Crosby, F. (1987). Studies of nurse practitioner effectiveness. *Nursing Research, 36*, 303–308.

45. Spitzer, W. O., Sacket, D. L., Sibley, J. C., et al. (1974). The Burlington randomized trial of the nurse practitioner. *New England Journal of Medicine, 290*, 251–256.

46. Billingsley, M. C., & Harper, D. C. (1982). The extinction of the nurse practitioner: Threat or reality? *Nurse Practitioner, 7*(9), 22–30.

47. American Nurses Association's first position on education for nursing. (1966). *American Journal of Nursing, 66*, 515.

48. Hsiao, V., & Edmunds, M. W. (1982). Master's vs CE: The debate continues. *Nurse Practitioner, 7*(10), 42–46.

49. American Nurses Association. (1985). *The scope of practice of the primary health care nurse practitioner.* Kansas City, MO: Author.

50. Bates, B. (1974). Twelve paradoxes: A message for nurse practitioners. *Nursing Outlook, 22*(11), 686–688.

51. Bicknell, W. J., Walsh, D. C., & Tanner, M. M. (1974). Substantive or decorative? Physicians' assistants and nurse practitioners in the United States. *Lancet, 7891*(2), 1241–1244.

2

SCOPE AND STANDARDS FOR ADVANCED PRACTICE NURSES

Elda G. Ramirez, MSN, RN, FNP, CS, CEN

Over the past century, nursing has been solidified as a highly regarded profession. A profession may be described by how it can be measured. Instinctively, nursing is a caring profession that cannot be measured in quantitative terms. The establishment of nursing as a profession defined some aspects to satisfy scientific and other professional communities. The registered nurse has a Nurse Practice Act, American Nurses Association, and a Board of Nurse Examiners that establishes rules and standards, follows through by review, and protects the profession. In addition, these governing bodies assist by establishing the profession's scope and standards of practice so that the individual nurse and other professions can identify the expanse of skill and knowledge for which the registered nurse is responsible and held attestable.

Advanced Practice

The advanced practice nurse (APN) is a registered nurse who has expanded the role into other dimensions of care. The first APNs were educated for specialized roles in the 1900s,[1] including nurses trained in anesthesia and tuberculosis management.[2] As time progressed, the clinical specialist or clinical nurse specialist (1940s) and the nurse practitioner (1960s) evolved.[1] It was not until the late 1970s and early 1980s that the term *advanced practice nurse* was coined to identify nurses who were specialized.[2] Today, APNs include clinical nurse specialists (CNSs), nurse practitioners (NPs), certified nurse anesthetists (CRNAs), and certified nurse midwives (CNMs).[2]

Taking the latter into consideration, it is imperative that APNs have delineated standards and scopes of practice. With the expansion of the nursing role, historically, other professions as well as administrations have needed clear delineations because the expanded role ebbs into other professional scopes of practice. To clarify further, the following terms have been defined.

Scope: extent of treatment, activity, or influence; synonym: range[3]

Scope of practice statements: what is legally allowable in each state under its nurse practice act; a guideline for the practice of nursing under special conditions and with advanced preparation[2]

Standard: something set up and established by authority as a rule for the measure of quantity, weight, extent, value, or quality[3]

Advanced practice nurse: application of an expanded range of practical, theoretical, and research-based therapeutics to phenomena experienced by patients within a specialized clinical area of the larger discipline of nursing[4]

Clinical nurse specialist: licensed registered nurse who has a graduate preparation as a CNS and is a clinical expert in theory-based and/or research-based nursing practice within a specialty area and does the following: integrates knowledge; designs, implements, and evaluates population-based programs of care; leads; consults; mentors; and serves as a change agent[5]

Nurse practitioner: a unique health care provider within the constellation of APNs. The NP assesses and manages both medical and nursing problems and does so by taking histories; conducting physical exams; ordering, performing, and interpreting appropriate diagnostic and laboratory tests; and prescribing pharmacological agents, treatment, and therapies for the conditions they diagnose[6]

Scope and Standards

The scope and standards for advanced practice nurses are established at the national level to encompass the basic parameters of the roles. The individual areas of specialty and individual states then further clarify what may or may not be included as a scope or standard for the area of specialty. The Emergency Nurses Association (ENA) has established position papers and a scope and standard of practice for APNs practicing in the emergency department. Professionals in the field of emergency care may use these as tools to establish the specific organizational specialty scope and standards.[7]

Blending the Roles

Although the roles of the CNS and the NP appear to be differentiated, in recent years they have started to blend. Some states offer regulation for all APNs without consideration of education as long as they have passed a national certification exam. Thus, the CNS and NP can be held to the same scope and standard of practice.[1] Other states no longer use the CNS role and extend the role of the NP into what was once that of the CNS. This has caused a great deal of debate because many believe the role of the NP is functional, whereas the role of the CNS is consultative and research generated or oriented toward nursing practice.[1] Therefore, the scope and standard of practice must be clear to the person who is practicing as an APN. In addition, the scope and standard for the specialty area and particular state and institution must be clearly defined for the employer.

The governing bodies that have provided the most recent information related to scope and standards of practice inquiries are

American Nurses Association (www.nursingworld.org)

American Academy of Nurse Practitioners (www.aanp.org)

National Association of Clinical Nurse Specialists (www.nacns.org)

Emergency Nurses Association (www.ena.org)

American College of Nurse Practitioners (www.nurse.org/acnp)

State Board of Nurse Examiners—organization based on state

National Council of State Boards of Nursing (www.ncsbn.org)

National League of Nursing (www.nln.org)

REFERENCES

1. Lynch, A. M. (1996). At the crossroads: We must blend the CNS + NP roles. *Online Journal of Issues in Nursing.* Retrieved from http://www.nursingworld.org/ojin/tpc1/tpc1_5.htm.
2. Hawkins, J. W., & Thibodeau, J. A. (2000). Advanced practice roles in nursing. In J. W. Hawkins & J. A. Thibodeau (Eds.), *The advanced practice nurse: Issues for the new millennium* (5th ed., pp. 7–40). New York: Springer.
3. *Merriam-Webster's Collegiate Dictionary.* (2002). [Electronic version]. Retrieved from http://www.m-w.com.
4. Hamric, A. B. (2000). A definition of advanced nursing practice. In A. B. Hamric, J. A. Spross, & C. M. Hanson (Eds.), *Advanced nursing practice: An integrative approach* (2nd ed., pp. 53–73). New York: W. B. Saunders.
5. National Association of Clinical Nurse Specialists. (1998). *NACNS statement on clinical nurse specialist practice and education.* Harrisburg, PA: Author.
6. American Academy of Nurse Practitioners. (1998). *Scope of practice for nurse practitioners.* Austin, TX: Author.

PART TWO

LEADERSHIP/ADMINISTRATION

3

ENTREPRENEURSHIP

Elisabeth K. Weber, RN, MA, CEN, CCNS

Just snap on the television in the middle of the night and you might think that anyone can be successful in business. There is no question that nurses are smart enough to be successful in any business venture, but just because you can become a nurse entrepreneur does not mean it is the right path for you. This chapter is designed to help you assess your potential for entrepreneurship, and if you chose to explore this opportunity, it provides an overview of recommendations for a successful business launch. Once you become a nurse entrepreneur with a successful thriving business, there are numerous additional resources for seeking advisors, support, and capital.

Certain skills have been identified that almost always ensure success in entrepreneurial ventures, with the range virtually unlimited. For the purposes of this chapter, we limit ourselves to the advanced practice nurse (APN) whose entrepreneurial venture is an outgrowth of his or her experience, education, and skills.

There are thought to be at least 4,000 nurse entrepreneurs in the United States, but there is no definitive source in which all nurse entrepreneurs are counted.[1] Peter Drucker reminds us, "Successful careers are not planned. They develop when people are prepared for opportunities because they know their strengths, their method of work, and their values. Knowing where one belongs can transform an ordinary person—hard working and competent but otherwise mediocre—into an outstanding performer."[2] White, a nurse entrepreneur, wrote, "One of my criteria for employment is that work has to be both fun and rewarding."[3] In most cases, fun and rewards spring from something for which we have a passion and in which we excel. As a nurse entrepreneur, you will assume more control over your employment and no longer live in fear of organizational restructuring or a philosophical or value mismatch. Entrepreneurship and full-time employment are not mutually exclusive. You can certainly utilize entrepreneurial innovations to enhance both professional and personal areas of life.

The Entrepreneurial Adventure

Everyone who seeks entrepreneurial experiences will approach them slightly differently. Just as in the nursing process, we begin with four areas of assessment that encompass the first steps for a nurse entrepreneur.

- Learning more about business principles and practices
- A self-assessment of talent and capabilities
- A market assessment of potential customers
- Determining if this will be a gradual or full-time entrepreneurial venture and determining how this will fit into your life

The first area, an understanding of business basics may be learned in a formal educational setting; by reading in the library, in bookstores, or online; or by taking workshops or joining business development groups. You need not get an MBA or become a business expert to be a successful nurse entrepreneur. Second, a self-assessment of your capabilities and talents should be completed prior to embarking on an entrepreneurial venture.[4] Schulmeister offers a number of questions that should be answered before starting a nurse consultation practice (Table 3-1).

Although you may have excellent business skills, if there are no unmet needs and no market demands, then even a spectacular business will fail. The concepts of entrepreneurial marketing, the

Table 3-1
Important Questions to Answer Before Starting a Nursing Consultation Practice
1. Why does starting a consultation practice interest me? Is this something I really want to do, or am I reacting to something else going on in my life?
2. What are my clinical strengths and areas in which growth is needed?
3. What are my personal strengths and areas in which growth is needed?
4. How well do I cope with uncertainty?
5. How essential is a steady income?
6. Do I have the necessary reserves (financial, emotional, physical) to cope if the business venture is a failure?
7. Do I have the support of those closest to me?
8. Do I have the time and energy required to get the business off the ground?
9. What sacrifices am I willing to make to devote time and attention to starting and growing the consultation business?

Reprinted from Schulmeister, L. (1999). Starting a nursing consultation practice. *Clinical Nurse Specialist, 13*(2), 94–100.

third point, will be discussed in greater depth later in this chapter.

The last area of assessment is to determine if this entrepreneurial venture will start gradually or as a full-time business. The gradual start may come from an unexpected opportunity or the sudden realization that you have specific skills that can be marketed. Often an opportunity to leave full-time employment opens up during an organizational redesign, or you may relocate due to family responsibilities with the option for self-employment suddenly available. It matters less how you begin and in what capacity than that you begin with a tentative plan and enough resources so that financial pressures do not stifle creativity and enthusiasm. Whether your money comes from full-time employment, part-time employment, a nest egg, or an inheritance, you will still require a financial plan.

Are motivation and an entrepreneurial spirit enough to sustain a successful business? Although many experts believe that passion and motivation[3,6,7,8,11,12] are the building blocks for the entrepreneur, a set of basic skills is also necessary for

the nurse entrepreneur to be successful. These skills begin with a state of mind. The nurse entrepreneur must first and foremost be self-motivated, self-directed, self-confident, and enthusiastic.[3,6,7,11,12] The nurse entrepreneur must also have expertise and skills in the area being marketed. Other skills of the successful nurse entrepreneur include organization, resourcefulness, great interpersonal skills, perseverance, and flexibility.[3,6,7,11,12] Papp best summarizes many authors by stating, "A successful entrepreneur must be truly interested in the work, believe in the service, and be highly motivated."[8]

Models of Nurse Entrepreneurial Businesses

There are a number of models of nursing entrepreneurial businesses that include consultation or service options:[8]

- Purchase of expertise or process consultation
- Writing procedures and programs
- Providing clinical services
- Providing training and educational programs
- Offering a comprehensive program
- Focusing on a specialty area
- Case management

Schulmeister describes the concept of collaboration between two disciplines, such as between a nurse and an attorney, in another variation of traditional models of collaboration. She goes on to discuss the opportunities for independent nursing consultation that exist in many of the following areas.[4]

- Patient advocacy
- Corporate wellness
- Child care
- Diabetic management
- Elder care
- Ethics
- Individual and family counseling
- Pain management

She notes an APN with expertise in internal consultation does not need to learn new skills but must apply these skills in a new setting, which is both the challenge and opportunity for nurse entrepreneurs.

Professional Image

As with most professional issues, quality in all one does will create favorable impressions.[8] A professional image may help you to get work and opportunities, but professional outcomes build your reputation. Depending on the type of business, you may want to either use your own name or develop a business image with another name or trademark. Your business concept should be clearly defined by this point. Business cards are a must for any nurse entrepreneur. I should stress that business cards sitting in a box do nothing to help you; they should be liberally distributed to anyone and everyone you know. Besides nursing colleagues and professional associates, you should distribute them to your neighbors, your college alumni association, your investment group, your book group, and church members who may know someone who can be a source of work. Business cards should be printed on good quality stock. Eventually you will need a logo for your business that you can apply to letterhead, brochures, and any other written material you produce.[10]

Business Planning

Every author who has written of a successful business venture has stressed that a business plan is necessary. To complete a business plan, attend a class or workshop, seek online support, buy a book that walks you through the process, or if your city is large enough, seek assistance from a small business or women's business development center. Business planning "forces you to respond to questions in writing . . . and gives an opportunity to organize thought and focus on specific ideas."[8] Smith believes that "every business requires the detailed thought and direction that go into a business plan."[11] The exercise of answering the questions and describing aspects of your proposed business is more important than the format of your business plan. If you are seeking funding from the government or other group, then the business plan must be detailed and explicit and conform to the rules of the money-granting entity. If you are utilizing your own skills and knowledge base in a consultative business, the business plan needs to be less comprehensive and detailed. When Bergman interviewed four nurse entrepreneurs, she concluded, "While a business plan may serve as the blueprint for your business, it is equally important to know you are not bound by your original plans and projections. A successful business plan is also flexible."[12] Drucker believes it is "rarely possible—or even particularly fruitful—to look too far ahead. A plan can usually cover no more than eighteen months and still be reasonably clear and specific."[2] One can never be certain what opportunity will present itself, and thus business planning remains at all times a work in progress.

Legal Issues

Do not neglect legal and accounting professional support because numerous nurse entrepreneurs wrote that legal advice was money well spent.[11,12,13] One way to lessen legal bills may be to work with a local law school's small business opportunity center.[14] One initial decision is whether a business will be a sole proprietorship, a partnership, or a corporation. Manthey believes that the time to incorporate is when it will reduce the amount of taxes you pay and/or when you want to reduce the risk of being personally sued.[9] There may be federal legal issues at tax time, state legal issues if your business is clinically driven, or local legal issues if you work out of your home. Adding employees to your business brings an entire new aspect of legal issues.

One caution, especially for those who are in a consultation business, is the aspect of intellectual property, or what Curtin and Simpson discuss as "intellectual capital . . . or what's in your head."[15] They write about the four types of intellectual property rights: (1) patents, (2) copyrights, (3) trade secrets, and (4) trademarks. Each affords a different type of legal protection. Table 3-2 provides a description for each of the intellectual property rights. Curtin and Simpson go on to say, "It seems that employers may indeed own what's in your head, even if you promise not to put it to use, at least for a period of time." Intellectual property is a major issue for nurse consultants.[9] It is always best to reach an agreement about product ownership before embarking on a business that sells it. It is worthwhile, then, for a nurse entrepreneur to be cognizant of protecting intellectual property while you are teaching or using it in your work. By learning the difference between

Table 3-2

	Types of Intellectual Property Rights
INTELLECTUAL PROPERTY RIGHT	DEFINITION
Patent	A 17-year exclusive monopoly on the right to make, use, and sell a qualifying invention
Copyright	A copyright merely protects the form in which ideas are expressed
Trade secret	A trade secret is any formula, pattern, compound, device process, tool or mechanism that is kept in secret and that gives its owner a competitive advantage
Trademark	A trademark protects the symbol or names used to distinguish products in the marketplace

the types of intellectual property you can protect yourself and avoid being sued for using someone else's intellectual property without permission.[9] As a career develops and ideas are generated, one can rarely be certain when a fact or process was truly learned. This makes it important to give credit to those team members who have assisted in successful process implementations. Rarely has anyone, save for solitary geniuses, developed something without the assistance of others. Thus, I stress the importance of seeking appropriate legal advice and representation as you become a nurse entrepreneur.

Financial Planning

There are several issues to consider within financial planning, and they include expenses, financing, and fee setting. One of the challenges is how to package and price knowledge and experience so that others will pay market-price fees for that service.[9] Even the best initial calculations of time can be underestimated when calculating the time needed to complete the project. One author recommends that other nurse consultants in the community be contacted and asked their rates, although they may not be willing to share this information. If one is able to obtain competing fees, then one can compare education and experience and then factor that into the rates. Setting fees that the market will bear is another method of determining what to charge.[4] The conclusion by a number of nurse entrepreneurs is that one must charge an hourly fee that will cover expenses and generate income. "Whenever possible, try to find out what your client expects to pay, how much

the client has allocated or has available, and what other consultants in this area of expertise are charging."[9]

It is important to have an amount of money available for living and business expenses, ranging for anywhere from 3 months to 1 year of expenses. Certainly the expenses are less for a home office for a consultation business than for another type of business, but one does not need to own every piece of office equipment if access to it is readily available at a local copy center, for example. Although there are many funding sources available, from personal savings to low-interest loans from family members, it is also common for nurse entrepreneurs to tap their own sources of credit and also to pursue small business loans through the Small Business Administration (www.sba.gov). Only you, your family, and your accountant and financial advisor can help determine where to obtain the money needed to start your business.

Market Analysis and Marketing

Determining the needs of your potential client can be completed through a process of market research, which begins with investigating the validity of your service with a trusted colleague. Making observations in the field and networking with as many people as possible and interviewing them about possible needs is important. You can also use questionnaires and surveys targeted to key people who may use your services and assess the competition by reviewing brochures and other promotional materials. This evaluation of your competitors may help identify opportunities to work cooperatively with the competition.[10]

Several nurse entrepreneurs describe the best marketing as word of mouth. It is helpful to spend time networking, writing, and speaking, for by becoming an expert, one is both marketing and assuring clients that they are getting a specific level of expertise for their money. For most nurse entrepreneurs, the product is the nurse because usually it is your own image, skills, knowledge, and interpersonal abilities that you market. Thus, for an entrepreneur, marketing is both promoting yourself and convincing others that you have something they need.

Buresh and Gordon write that all nurses should be prepared to take advantage of openings so that we can respond constructively, even when disheartening comments about nursing are verbalized. Nurse entrepreneurs are at a disadvantage in some cases when the general public does not have a true understanding of the scope of nursing.[16] Are nurse entrepreneurs in nursing or business? A clear and concise answer to this question will help you to market your business.

Advice from the Experts

If the length of this chapter were unlimited, it would be a treat to have a wide range of successful nurse entrepreneurs give you their best "lessons learned." Because that is impossible in this format, I refer additional interested readers to a book called *How I Became a Nurse Entrepreneur: Tales from 50 Nurses in Business,* a book published by the National Nurses in Business Association. The first-person stories are enlightening and, besides hearing directly from your entrepreneurial colleagues, are the next best thing to help you avoid your own entrepreneurial detours.

Marie Manthey provides a note of caution for all budding entrepreneurs. She writes, "Beware of the tendency to spend a lot of time and energy creating the perfect package/product representation of your expertise. I think it is far more important to spend that time listening to the field, discerning the need, and figuring out how to package your expertise to meet that need than to create the perfect representation of your service."[9]

Challenges to Success

The major challenges to success as a nurse entrepreneur include keeping focused, staying connected, locating resources, and controlling expenses.[17] Staying focused implies a regular time and place for work and a balance of completing work and seeking additional work. Staying connected implies continuously networking and maintaining professional connections. Locating resources implies both the resources for obtaining work and the resources to complete the work. The challenge of controlling expenses remains in the forefront because few of us can work for the sheer joy of the work. There is a clear recognition that the success or failure of this entrepreneurial venture is based on one's own abilities. Like a roller coaster, which provides both sheer terror and amazing fun, a well-planned and executed entrepreneurship allows unlimited opportunities for creativity and innovation. May you become a leader in the concept of "disruptive innovation," as described by Christensen in the *Harvard Business Review.*[18] Disrupting the current health care model as a leader while utilizing entrepreneurial principles may offer a fundamental mechanism through which we will build a higher quality, more convenient, and lower cost health system. May you find luck and success in your entrepreneurial ventures.

REFERENCES

1. Zagury, C. S. (2001). *Nurse entrepreneur: Building the bridge of opportunity.* Long Branch, NJ: Vista Publishing.
2. Drucker, P. (1999). Managing oneself. *Harvard Business Review, 77*(2), 64–74.
3. White, J. (2000). Clinical nurse specialist entrepreneur: Getting started. *Clinical Nurse Specialist, 14*(2), 49–50.
4. Schulmeister, L. (1999). Starting a nursing consultation practice. *Clinical Nurse Specialist, 13*(2), 94–100.
5. Hilton, J. (1999). Doing your own thing. *Nursing Standard, 14*(3), 77.
6. Collinson, G. (2000). Encouraging the growth of the nurse entrepreneur. *Professional Nurse, 15*(6), 365–367.
7. Kowal, N. (1998). Specialty practice entrepreneur: The advanced practice nurse. *Nursing Economic$, 16*(5), 277–278.
8. Papp, E. (2000). Starting a business as a nurse consultant. *AAOHN Journal, 48*(3), 136–142.
9. Manthey, M. (1999). Financial management for entrepreneurs. *Nursing Administration Quarterly, 23*(4), 81–85.

10. Czaplewski, L. (1999). Marketing your expertise. *Journal of Intravenous Nursing, 22*(2), 75–80.

11. Smith, W. (2000). Setting up a home-based business. *American Journal of Nursing, 100*(2), 22.

12. Bergmann, P. (1998). Invest in yourself. Lessons learned from nurse entrepreneurs. *Nursing Forum, 33*(3), 17–21.

13. Kuric, J. (1999). Me, an entrepreneur? *SCI Nursing, 16*(4), 133–134.

14. Kaiser, R. (2002, June 12). Law schools offer less expensive source of legal advice. *Chicago Tribune,* Section 3, p. 4.

15. Curtin L., & Simpson, R. (1999). Who owns your ideas? *Health Management Technology, 20*(6), 38–39.

16. Buresh, B., & Gordon, S. (2000). *From silence to voice: What nurses know and must communicate to the public.* Ontario, Canada: Canadian Nurses Association.

17. Schulmeister, L. (1999). The challenges of a home-based nursing consultation business. *Clinical Nurse Specialist, 13*(2), 101–103.

18. Christensen, C., Bohmer, R., & Kenagy, J. (2000). Will disruptive innovations cure health care? *Harvard Business Review, 78*(5), 102–112.

4 REIMBURSEMENT

Marlene Angelico, RN, MSN, ANP

For the past few years, change has been a constant for our nation's health care system, most notably in reimbursement practices. There has also been a rising trend in health care costs and premiums. Emergency department (ED) advanced practice nurses (APNs) have become solid participants in the reimbursement process while providing cost-effective health care. Most health care bills in the United States are paid by managed care plans and insurance companies with provision for direct reimbursement to the practitioner. This chapter will discuss the various types of reimbursement that are available to the APN, barriers to the reimbursement process, and the process of credentialing with provider panels to obtain direct payment. The Medicare and Medicaid programs will be briefly discussed in relation to APN reimbursement and fraud, and a concise synopsis of third-party payers will be presented. Although most of the information in this chapter pertains to APNs in general, there are specific state regulations that pertain strictly to nurse practitioners (NPs) alone, and they will be noted when indicated. It is important for all APNs to become familiar with the reimbursement laws of their individual states as well as federal laws regarding reimbursement.

Types of APN Reimbursement

When it comes to payment for services, APNs do not have the same options as physicians. State and federal laws require Medicare, Medicaid, indemnity insurers, and managed care plans to reimburse physicians for their services. APNs have the same potential for reimbursement, but some insurers refuse to pay for the same services from an APN that would be reimbursed if performed by a physician. When an APN is unable to bill for services rendered, the APN loses the ability to demonstrate financial productivity.[1] This can be devastating to the APN's practice.

Individual payers, namely Medicare, Medicaid, managed care organizations, and indemnity insurers, each have their own reimbursement policies and fee schedules; each operates under a separate body of law. Some payers will reimburse APNs in the same manner as they reimburse physicians, whereas other payers have specific policies pertaining to APN reimbursement. However, every company will not reimburse every APN for services.[2] This diversity is the root of much confusion among APNs and billing service departments. It is the responsibility of the APN, along with the financial officer of the employing organization, to obtain the specific reimbursement policy and reimbursement schedule for each organization billed for services.

Direct reimbursement, or payment designated specifically to an APN for services rendered, is the optimal type of reimbursement. APNs and health care organizations should strive for direct reimbursement by fighting for improved legislation that would guide all health care reimbursement organizations toward direct reimbursement for APNs. Direct reimbursement can come from Medicare, Medicaid, private insurance payers, or managed care organizations. Direct reimbursement can be facilitated by listing APNs in provider directories, which gives consumers an expanded choice of health care providers. In addition, this reinforces the recognition of APNs as direct providers.

In 1997, the Balanced Budget Act (BBA) was signed, which enabled APNs in all geographic and practice settings to receive direct Medicare reimbursement at 85% of the prevailing physician rate. This represented the greatest adjustment to Medicare since its inception in 1965.[3] The law became effective January 1, 1998.

Before the law was enacted, Medicare reimbursement to APNs was fragmented and cumbersome, and payment was sporadic. As a matter of fact, before the BBA, APNs received Medicare reimbursement in rural areas and skilled nursing facilities only.[4] The successful passage of the BBA was the result of persistent, effective lobbying by APN organization representatives. It resulted in inclusion of APN reimbursement language into the BBA.

Barriers to Reimbursement

Reimbursement remains an issue for APNs across the nation, although it is no longer an impossible feat. Direct reimbursement for an APN's services and being listed on provider panels continue to be goals in the quest for reimbursement.

In many cases, recognition for an APN's services comes straight from the collaborating physician.[5] Oftentimes, practices welcome the cost-effective, efficient care, but some insurance plans remain disinterested and do not accept APNs on their provider panel for reimbursement. A study conducted in New York indicated that approximately 60% of third-party payers do not credential nurse practitioners (NPs) to be on their provider panels.[5]

An ED APN may be working as a silent, rather than as a recognized, provider. In essence, an APN may not be receiving due recognition for services rendered. Consequently, the results of revenue generation and productivity are buried in grouped numbers, which may leave one vulnerable when an organization cuts costs.[6] It is important for APNs to be listed as direct providers on insurance panels because productivity and revenue generation can be reviewed. Moreover, the role becomes more visible and legitimized.[6]

An additional barrier to APN reimbursement is the public's lack of understanding concerning their role and scope of practice. Promotion of the role of the NP in the media and by other health care providers could increase consumer knowledge, thereby providing them with an additional choice in their health care provider. Consumer approval and satisfaction with the role of the APN might prompt payers such as Medicare and private insurers to add them to their provider directories.

Finally, reimbursement laws can be confusing for providers, carriers, and consumers. This, in itself, can be a barrier to reimbursement.

Credentialing for Provider Panels

For the APN to be reimbursed for services, she or he must first be credentialed and included on an insurer's provider panel. Because direct payment of APNs by third-party payers is essential to the long-term financial strength of nursing practice,[7] all APNs should seek credentialing within their practice institution and their reimbursement agencies to facilitate reimbursement.

Credentialing involves an application process which includes the collection of educational, licensing, malpractice, employment, and certification data on each provider.[2] The objective is to determine if the applicant is adequately prepared to care for the patient and, thus, to be granted reimbursement privileges. For a complete overview of the credentialing process, see Chapter 21.

Third-party payers differ in their standards and guidelines for credentialing and admission to their provider panels. Each payer has their own forms and policies for credentialing, contracting, and reimbursing providers. Moreover, the requirements of a particular payer may vary from state to state. The APN provider should contact the third-party payer to request information regarding credentialing criteria and a credentialing form.

Medicare Reimbursement

The Medicare system was created in 1965 and is composed of two programs, Medicare Part A and Medicare Part B. Medicare Part A covers hospitalization, skilled nursing facilities, and some home health services. Medicare Part B covers the services of physicians, APNs, and other Medicare health care providers. Part B also covers outpatient hospital services and laboratory and diagnostic services.[8] The Centers for Medicare and Medicaid Services (CMS), formerly named the Health Care Financing Administration (HCFA), is the agency that administers Medicare.

An ED APN may be reimbursed on a fee-for-service basis after obtaining a Medicare provider number or personal identification number (PIN), an important first step to being in the loop for reimbursement. Call the Medicare carrier in your area and request an application for a PIN. When a PIN is obtained, Medicare may be billed for reimbursable services. "NP's may bill Medicare Part B for services which would be physician services if performed by a physician, but which are performed by an NP."[8] To be reimbursed, ED APNs must use their own PIN. If the bill meets the criteria, Medicare will reimburse at 85% of the physician rate. If the requested reimbursement fee does not meet Medicare's definition of a "physician service," it will not be reimbursed.[8] In addition, services that are within the realm of nursing will not be covered under Part B.[8] For a list of noncovered services, the local Medicare carrier should be contacted.

Medicare has strict rules qualifying an APN for reimbursement. An APN must hold a state license and be certified by a national certifying body. Effective January 2003, an APN applying for a Medicare number must possess a master's degree, as well as state licensure and national certification. As Buppert[8] summarized, Medicare will reimburse NPs under the following conditions.

1. The NP meets Medicare qualification requirements;
2. The facility will accept 85% of the physician fee schedule, submitted under the NP provider number;
3. The services performed are "physician services" or those for which a physician can bill Medicare;
4. The services are performed in collaboration with a physician;
5. The services are within the NP's scope of practice as defined in state law; and
6. No other facility or other provider either charges or is paid with respect to the furnishing of services.[8]

The "Incident To" concept will be discussed briefly because it is frequently referred to, but it is usually not applicable to ED patients. "Incident To" is a Medicare phrase that describes a concept involving billing incident to a physician's services. With this ruling, a physician may bill under his or her own provider number for the services performed by a nonphysician provider with whom he or she is employed or has a contractual relationship.[9] "Incident To" is primarily used in an office setting, is limited to follow-up care, and requires that a physician be on-site. When services are provided in the emergency department, the service should be billed under the provider number of the rendering clinician, whether it is an APN or a physician.[9]

Medicare Fraud

The HCFA has developed strictly enforced rules for Medicare patients. APNs as well as physicians who do not follow the rules can be charged with Medicare fraud.[8]

When Congress authorized payments to APNs for Medicare patients with the passage of the BBA, it created a new source of reimbursement and a potential for liability. It is the responsibility of the APN to be aware of the billing practices for their services. Failure to follow Medicare billing rules can result in fines, payment denial, fraud prosecution, loss of Medicare billing ability, and loss of employment.[10] Guidelines to follow for avoiding Medicare fraud are outlined in Table 4-1.

If an APN is unclear on billing procedures, the practice or hospital compliance officer should be contacted. A Medicare carrier or private attorney who specializes in Medicare reimbursement can

Table 4-1
Guidelines to Avoid Medicare Fraud[8]
1. Physician practices that employ NPs must coordinate billing to avoid seeking duplicate payments.
2. The services performed and billed by the NP must be within the NP's scope of practice.
3. Services that are billed for must be rendered and documented.
4. A hospital cannot bill for an NP's services if the hospital receives reimbursement for the NP's salary from Medicare under the cost report (Medicare Part A).

be an additional resource for advice to avoid Medicare fraud.[8]

Medicaid Reimbursement

Medicaid rules do not echo Medicare rules. Medicaid is jointly funded by state and federal governments. In most situations, the activity of Medicaid is controlled by the state. "Medicaid is available to anyone who can demonstrate need as established through income and asset standards, and is either a child, has dependent children, is pregnant, blind, disabled and age 65 or more."[11]

State regulations vary in the billing of an APN's services. Under current law, state Medicaid programs are required to provide direct reimbursement to certified nurse midwives, pediatric NPs, and family NPs.[12] Some states may broaden this law to include APNs in other specialties, who then may receive Medicaid reimbursement to the extent permitted by state law.[12]

To be accepted as a Medicaid provider, one must apply to the state Medicaid agency. Reimbursement may be more complicated if the Medicaid patient is also covered by a managed care organization (MCO). To obtain reimbursement for a Medicaid patient enrolled in an MCO, the APN must also be admitted to the provider panel of the specific MCO. Reimbursement by Medicaid is generally lower than that paid by a commercial insurer.

Following acceptance to the Medicaid provider panel, one will receive a Medicaid provider number. The Medicaid agency may be billed on an HCFA 1500 form. Reimbursement amounts differ from state to state. In some states, Medicaid will reimburse an APN from 70% to 100% of the physician fee.[2] State law controls the reimbursement rate.

As with Medicare, all providers are expected to follow Medicaid's rules. Claims are monitored, and providers are expected to be familiar with the rules. Providers that are suspected of fraud are subject to investigation and fines. For specific questions on Medicaid reimbursement, contact the state Medicaid agency, or go online at http://cms.hhs.gov/medicaid/default.asp.

Additional Third-Party Payers

An MCO is an umbrella term that may include health maintenance organizations (HMOs), preferred provider organizations (PPOs), and physician-sponsored organizations (PSOs). These MCOs provide payment for the services as well as the health care services.

Not all MCOs will admit APNs to their provider panels. The MCO may assume that the physician is responsible for the care provided, although the care may actually have been provided by an APN. The services of an APN will not be fully recognized by a managed care plan unless they are allowed direct billing privileges for services they have provided.[13]

Many MCO contracts are silent on delegation, and some contracts will require a specific primary care provider to furnish services. As a rule, APNs in the ED do not need to apply to MCO panels because they are not seeking primary care status. Some MCO contracts will allow an APN to be reimbursed in some states, but not in others. The policy on providers is up to the individual state.

An indemnity insurer or commercial insurer pays for medical care on a fee-for-service basis to health care providers. These insurers have their own fee structure, but their fee schedule is generally based on "usual and customary" charges.[8] Reimbursement policies vary with these payers, but ordinarily they do not credential APNs to receive direct reimbursement.

Conclusion

APNs remain among the most cost-effective providers of care in EDs and clinics. With their independent licensure, experience, and education, they are qualified to provide a wide range of services. For an APN to have the opportunity to participate in the delivery of health care in the ED, the APN must first become knowledgeable regarding the reimbursement process.

The best plan for reimbursement is to comply with established rules. Get credentialed by insurers that provide billing numbers to APNs. If billing under your own provider number for direct reimbursement, be certain there is documentation supporting the service that was billed. If seeking direct reimbursement, one should personally provide the billed service.[14]

Recognizing APN services in payment systems is important to maintaining accessibility of APN services, examining outcomes of advanced practice nursing, and ensuring fiscal accountability.[4] As Sullivan-Marx et al.[4] reported, "Payment is society's overt recognition of a professional group's authority to practice." Recognition as direct providers for health care services is a pivotal victory for APNs. We must pursue and cultivate this achievement by exploring the systems used to establish payment and fee schedules to ensure that APNs continue to provide services that have an impact on the quality of care.

REFERENCES

1. Buppert, C. (2001). What information can you give me about independent NP practices? *Medscape Nurses, 3*(1). Retrieved December 23, 2002 from www.medscape.com/viewarticle/413411

2. Buppert, C. (1999). Reimbursement for nurse practitioner services. In *Nurse practitioner's business practice and legal guide* (pp. 252–267). Gaithersburg, MD: Aspen.

3. Sullivan-Marx, E. (1998). Medicare reimbursement for advanced practice nurses: In the front door! *Nursing Outlook, 46*(1), 40–41.

4. Sullivan-Marx, E., Happ, M. B., Bradley, K., & Maislin, G. (2000). Nurse practitioner services: Content and relative work value. *Nursing Outlook, 48*(6), 269–275.

5. Herrick, T. (2002). The pulse of managed care in 2002: A look at rising costs, reimbursement impanelment, and provider directories. *Clinician News, 6,* 1, 10–11.

6. Shay, L. E. (2001). Provider and physician: Title use in HMO provider panels. *Nurse Practitioner, 26*(3), 71–74.

7. Swan, B. A. (2000). Perspectives in ambulatory care. Credentialing, contracting, and reimbursing nurse practitioners. *Nursing Economics, 18*(5), 267–270.

8. Buppert, C. (2002). Billing for nurse practitioner services: Guidelines for NPs, physicians, employers, and insurers. *Medscape Nurses, 4*(1). Retrieved December 23, 2002 from www.medscape.com/viewarticle/422935

9. Buppert, C. (2002). Billing physician services provided by NPs in a hospital. *The Green Sheet, 4*(3). Retrieved December 23, 2002 from www.medscape.com/viewarticle/431137

10. Buppert, C. (2001). Avoiding Medicare fraud. Part 1. *Nurse Practitioner, 26*(1), 70–75.

11. Illinois Department of Public Aid. What is Medicaid? Retrieved December 23, 2002 from http://www.state.il.us/dpa/html/medicaid.htm

12. Patykula, J. M. (1999). Update on reimbursement issues faced by neonatal nurse practitioners. *Neonatal Networks, 18*(8), 41–43.

13. Abood, S., & Franklin, P. (2000). Why care about Medicare reimbursement? *American Journal of Nursing, 100*(6), 69–72.

14. Reading, N. L. (2002). Coding strategies for NPs. *Advance for Nurse Practitioners, 10*(2), 22–23.

5

CASE MANAGER ROLE IN THE EMERGENCY DEPARTMENT

Sharon Schultz, RN, BS, MPH, CCPSI

With increasing volumes of emergency patients that currently exceed 108 million[1] and hospital admissions increasing by 14% in 1997 alone,[2] the urgency for initiatives to explore more efficient and cost-effective ways to manage health care delivery is essential. Decreasing reimbursement from both state and federal agencies, capitated contracts, and whatever comes next will continue to force hospital administrators to demand new and innovative ways to deliver high-quality, timely care with less resource consumption. In an effort for hospitals to stay financially solvent, the current costly management of medical and nursing care must be reviewed and reinvented. In the past, the physician has been central to directing the "what, when, and where" for treatments, procedures, and testing. But it is the nurse who directly affects the total care of the patient and the family. This isn't just anyone's work; this is nursing's work. Nursing care is the only constant in the patient visit, whether it is an inpatient, emergency, or outpatient encounter. It is the nurse who not only coordinates the care, treatments, and procedures for the patient, but it is also the nurse who ensures the environment of healing from hospital to home. Nurses have an incredible opportunity to make a tremendous difference in the delivery of health care by using advanced practice nurses (APNs) in the role of case managers (CMs).[3] The challenge for the APN in the emergency department (ED) is to demonstrate the importance of the CM role in this very diverse setting.

This chapter will define case management and the roles and responsibilities of ED APN CMs and share successful ED case management models. APNs are encouraged to think of this chapter as a recipe, one that encourages the APN to take a few ingredients from some of the experts, add a few individualized ideas, and create a role that will meet one's professional goals.

What Is Case Management?

The American Nurses Association defines case management as a "dynamic and systematic collaborative approach to providing and coordinating health care services to a defined population. It is a participative process to identify and facilitate options and services for meeting individuals' health needs, while decreasing fragmentation and duplication of care and enhancing quality, cost effective clinical outcomes."[4] In other words, the CM assesses the needs of patients, either individually or in a cohort, collaborates with the medical team to outline an explicit and competent treatment plan, sees that this plan is implemented in the most explicit and accurate manner using cost-effective techniques, and then evaluates this treatment, reporting the results back to the team. Of particular importance to the CM is analyzing and changing systems of care delivery in an effort to make the system of care more responsive to individual needs. To accomplish this, the CM needs to adopt a responsible economic posture as well as impeccable ethical standards.[5] An example of one CM's workload is provided in Figure 5-1.

Why Do We Need CMs?

Data from the 1997 Healthcare Cost and Utilization Project, a federal-state-industry partnership representing hospitals across the United States, list 14 reasons why APNs should focus on case management in the ED (see Table 5-1).[6] While reviewing these findings, the APN can quickly identify target populations that consume the most resources and finances from the ED. The CM can use this information to better focus on trends in

FIGURE 5-1 *Communicating Workload*

EMERGENCY DEPARTMENT ADVANCE PRACTICE RN CM PRODUCTIVITY MONTHLY REPORT

Name: _____

Month:	Jan	Feb	Mar	Apr	May	June	July	Aug	Sep	Oct	Nov	Dec
# of total cases emergency patients reviewed												
# of total emergency patients case managed												
# of emergency patients discharged to home with assistance												
# of emergency patients admitted to the hospital												
# of emergency patients referred to home health												
# of emergency patients referred to VNA												
# of emergency patients denied admission												
# of emergency patients denied case management												
# of emergency Level 2 cases managed (1 hr) Avg. estimated savings this month												
# of emergency Level 3 cases managed (3–4 hrs) Avg. estimated savings this month												
# of emergency Level 4 cases managed (3–4 hrs) Avg. estimated savings this month												
# of emergency Level 5 cases managed (2–3 hrs) Avg. estimated savings this month												
Total hours logged this month												
Total estimated $ $ $ saved this month												
Productivity ratio: Total hours per month/Total cases managed												
Variance codes used this month												
Comments:												

Reprinted with permission from Rush-Copley Medical Center, Aurora, IL, Emergency Department Case Management Productivity Tool, 2002.

Table 5-1	
Admissions Through the Emergency Department[6]	

- Five of the top 10 conditions for which people are admitted through the ED are related to heart problems.
- Two of the top 10 conditions are infectious: Pneumonia and septicemia.
- Pneumonia accounts for nearly 6% of all admissions through the ED.
- Nearly 55% of hospital stays for the very old (80 years and older) start in the ED, compared with 45% for younger age groups.
- 33% of all hospital admissions begin in the ED.
- Over 50% of all hospitalized patients have at least one comorbidity. Another 33% of patients have two or more comorbid factors.
- Drug abuse, psychoses, and depression are present as top 10 comorbidities for adolescents and adults up to age 44.
- Alcohol abuse is a top 10 comorbidity for adults ages 18 to 44.
- Infant respiratory distress is the most expensive condition treated in the hospital, with an average charge of $68,000.
- Two of the top 10 most expensive conditions are traumas:
  - Spinal cord injury ($53,000) and burns ($34,000).
- Government (Medicare and Medicaid) is billed for over half (54%) of all hospital stays.
- About 17% of the U.S. population is uninsured, and about 5% of all hospital patients are uninsured.
- Nearly 20% of hospitalizations for alcohol-related mental disorders and 23% of hospitalizations for substance abuse are uninsured patients.
- Over one third of all hospital admissions are through the ED.

health care utilization to reduce costs and improve patient care and customer satisfaction.

The Role of the APN CM in the ED

The CM should be proficient in organizational, professional, and interpersonal skills. Because it is essential that all APNs have a minimum of a graduate-level education, the CM brings a wealth of rich knowledge, critical-thinking abilities, and experience to the role. The CM is expected to use these skills to work autonomously while interacting with multiple professionals both within and outside the organization. This knowledge and experience is invaluable because the CM is expected to function in a role that is often ambiguous.[7]

Case management in the ED is different from other areas of care, in that the CM is not following just one or two patient types in a 12-hour shift, but may be involved with at least 40% of all the patients presenting to the ED. In addition, these patients are not followed for days but rather for hours, requiring the CM to have expert knowledge that is quickly accessible and sharp

organizational skills that can expedite care in a swift and competent manner. Knowing what resources are available to emergency patients within the hospital and community is a valuable asset for the CM.

Leadership is a key role for the CM. The CM assumes responsibility and accountability for the clinical management of ED patients requiring admission, transfer, or discharge to the community. The CM often leads a team consisting of other health professionals such as RNs, discharge planners, physical therapists, and social workers. The goal of the team is to improve clinical and financial performance in the ED.

The CM also needs to have a strong command of the nursing process and be able to integrate this process with the ED population targeted. The nursing process utilized by the CM includes[8]

- Assessment: Through the collection of comprehensive data provides integration of information from a wide variety of sources to make clinical judgments and decisions about appropriate recommendations and treatments.

- Diagnosis: Determines the diagnosis through critical analysis of assessment data.
- Outcome identification: Expected outcomes are derived from the assessment data and evidence-based guidelines. The expected outcomes are then communicated to the patient, family, and health care team.
- Planning: A comprehensive plan of care is developed, inclusive of interventions, treatments, and procedures, to attain expected outcomes shared with the health care team.
- Implementation: Interventions, treatments, and procedures are implemented, prescribed, or ordered to support and meet the expected outcomes.
  - Caring: Creates a compassionate and therapeutic environment with the aim of promoting comfort and preventing suffering.
  - Case management/coordination of care: Comprehensive clinical coordination of care and case management is provided.
  - Consultation: Provides consultation to influence the plan of care for patients, enhance the abilities of others, and effect change in the system.
  - Health promotion, health maintenance, and health teaching: Promotes complex strategies, interventions, and teaching to preserve and improve health and to prevent illness and injury.
  - Prescriptive authority and treatment: Use of prescriptive authority, procedures, and treatments, must be in accordance with state and federal laws and regulations, to treat illness and improve functional health status or to provide preventive care.
  - Referral: The need for additional care is identified and referrals and appointments are made.
- Evaluation: Progress toward goal and expected outcomes is evaluated against variances and guidelines.
  - Qualitative data such as patient and nurse satisfaction is one example of an excellent source of quality indicators.
  - Fiscal management: Provides data to demonstrate productivity, cost-effective care, and benchmark quality.[9]

Table 5-2 is an example of competency for the role of the CM that is provided under a framework developed by del Bueno et al.[10] focusing on the unique interpersonal dimension, technical,

Table 5-2		
Dimensions of Competent Performance of the APN CM		
Emergency Department Advanced Practice Registered Nurse (APRN) CM		
INTERPERSONAL DIMENSION	TECHNICAL SKILLS	CRITICAL THINKING
<ul><li>Strategizes solutions with the team on care and service opportunities</li><li>Able to stand alone; will not shirk from responsibility</li><li>Clearly and accurately articulates changes</li><li>Is approachable and easy to talk to</li><li>Responds to health care team members', patients', families', and payers' requests in a timely manner</li><li>Concepts are shared</li><li>Structures team meetings in a manner that is productive and results oriented</li></ul>	<ul><li>Benchmarks against highest achieving organizations on evidence-based practices, financial achievements, and outcomes management</li><li>Takes actions when there are unexpected variances</li><li>Takes actions to stay in compliance with all regulatory agencies</li><li>Coordinates regular clinical rounds with nurses</li><li>Implements best clinical practices that are "team" approved</li></ul>	<ul><li>Designs services across the continuum to ensure a seamless integration of services and care</li><li>Facilitates appropriate patient information to providers</li><li>Evaluates physician and nursing admitting patterns to expedite patient flow</li><li>Evaluates variances against expected outcomes</li><li>Synthesizes financial information and clinical outcomes to ensure appropriate delivery of care</li><li>Develops care guidelines for maximum results</li></ul>

Adapted from Porter-O'Grady, T., & Krueger Wilson, C. (1995). *The leadership revolution in health care: Altering systems, changing behavior.* Gaithersburg, MD: Aspen.

and critical-thinking skills that are integrated into each situation facing the CM. This example gives a clear picture of the CM role using criteria set forth by O'Grady and Krueger-Wilson in their book *The Leadership Revolution in Health Care*.[11]

Outcomes Management

CM models use outcomes management as the hallmark to their success. Outcomes management, put simply, is how one measures the achievement of goals. One of the most noticeable measurements in outcomes management is cost. For example, if one of the CM's goals is to reduce the cost of care for patients diagnosed with pneumonia, one of the strategies to reach this goal may be to reduce the number of sputum specimens obtained from patients. This alone will make a major difference in the cost for each patient and will be one way to demonstrate achievement of one particular goal. The following objectives of outcomes management in case management create new possibilities for the relationship between quality of care and cost of care: (1) achievement of expected or standardized outcomes; (2) promotion of collaborative practice, coordinated care, and continuity of care; (3) promotion of appropriate or reduced utilization of resources; (4) pro-

motion of professional development and satisfaction among nurses; (5) facilitation of testing, treatments, and procedures in the ED and (6) facilitation of home services to avert an admission.

The use of evidence-based research tools can help provide the CM with the information needed to make competent decisions.[12] Some of the evidence-based practice research tools are described in Table 5-3.

Strong teams need to be built for outcomes management to work. These teams often consist of physicians, nurses, social workers, therapists, those in utilization review roles, in-house case managers, finance staff, and administrators. The CM must be able to dialogue with colleagues about individual patients and to delineate patient needs in terms of functional status; physical, emotional, and psychological status; support systems; and financial status.

If the CM is to be successful in this role, she or he needs to have a clear understanding of how to manage care in the ED, how to evaluate data on costs, current APCs (Medicare Outpatient Prospective Payment System/Ambulatory Patient Classifications), International Classification of Diseases (ICD-9) codes, Medicare and Medicaid

Table 5-3	
Evidence-Based Practice Research Tools	
Critical pathways/ critical paths	■ Clinical management tools that organize, sequence, and time the major interventions of nursing staff, physicians, and other departments for a particular case type, subset, or condition
Clinical practice guidelines	■ The National Academy of Sciences' Institute of Medicine, Washington, D.C., adopted this term to refer to standards developed to assist practitioner and patient decisions about appropriate interventions in specific clinical circumstances
Practice parameters	■ The American Medical Association refers to practice parameters as educational tools that enable physicians to obtain the advice of recognized clinical experts, stay abreast of the latest clinical research, and assess the clinical significance of often-conflicting research findings
CareMaps®	■ Are elaborate critical pathways that show the relationship of sets of interventions to sets of intermediate outcomes along a time line ■ Merge standards of care with standards of practice in a cause-and-effect relationship across time[13] ■ Provide a means to measure appropriateness of clinical and financial outcomes when procedures are eliminated, variances in practices are limited or removed, collaboration in care is interdisciplinary, and the patient and family are involved in attaining goals for healing[14]

reimbursement codes, ED charges, payer mix, and profitability. Developing partnerships with the ED manager or a person who knows the charge master best, a medical records coder, a fiscal auditor, and a physician billing representative will make the job easier from the start. This information can help guide the CM on how to best manage costs, as well as to direct focus to the greatest financial and outcome variances. It will also give the physicians and staff access to financial information that they may not have known; this alone may help to decrease resource utilization.

Tools Necessary for Success

It is helpful for CMs to develop a list of tools necessary to be successful in their role. The following section will describe several tools this author has found helpful.

Emergency Department Case Management Plan

- Identify current APCs utilized.
- Provide education to nursing staff on documentation needed to validate nursing care, and evaluate daily until staff is proficient at capturing the essence of the care they provide.
- Simplify the task by limiting the number of patients to be managed. First, choose by consensus of the team; try to choose the patients most critical for a quick return on investment. This will help demonstrate the CM's value to leadership early on.[15] Take those patients and look at the cost versus reimbursement. If the cost is close to or exceeds reimbursement, start to investigate what is included and if there are any changes to be made. These patients should be frequent users of the ED or admissions.
- Next, design an interdisciplinary team that will develop criteria, guidelines, or CareMaps® to stay the course.
- Finally, carefully document outcomes of these interventions. Be sure to document cost, quality, and efficiency data.

Variance Tracking

A variance tracking tool is used for reporting the variances in care and costs of a given population or disease targeted for the CM to manage (Figure

---

FIGURE 5-2 *Variance Tracking Tool*

I. Prehospital Clinical Variance
Prehospital delay in treatment/procedure ☐
Prehospital medication error/complication ☐

II. Provider Clinical Variance
Diagnostic test unrelated to documented diagnosis ☐
Abnormal test not addressed in medical record ☐
Readmission for same diagnosis < 31days ☐
Life-threatening complication of sedation analgesia ☐
Postoperative complication ☐
Unexpected procedural complication ☐
Readmission within 31 days with (complication) related to previous emergency visit or admission ☐
Other ☐

III. Disposition Variance
Home health/visiting nurse delay ☐
Unable to take care of self ☐
Other ☐

IV. Patient/Family Variance
Patient/family refuse discharge ☐
Patient noncompliant with treatment regimen ☐
Unable to contact any caregivers ☐
Other ☐

V. Treatment Variance
Does not meet admission criteria ☐
Clinical guidelines not followed ☐
Missed home health/visiting nurse treatment/therapy ☐
Other ☐

VI. System Variance
Delay in OR schedule ☐
Delay due to weekend _____ ☐
Admission due to medication/procedure/ treatment/error ☐
Other ☐

Reprinted with permission from Rush-Copley Medical Center, Aurora, IL, 2002.

5-2). This tool will document productivity and aid in producing monthly reports, which should be shared with the organization's leadership team. It is important to share data with others on why some patients are in the hospital longer than others, why some patients can fit perfectly into an established care guideline, why some fall out, and the reasons that the length of stay can be so variable. Variance screens help document and track facts, revealing different reasons that lead to the unpredictability in patient outcomes, costs, and delays in discharge. Variability has a major cause and effect on escalating health care costs, whether it is related to a delay in service, nurse staffing, or an unexpected response to a treatment. Conveying variance information to all of the stakeholders helps to drive decisions on program development and eliminations.

Models of Success

Because case management focuses on the whole person, family, and community, and not just the episode of the illness or injury, several models are available to replicate illustrating the CM role in the ED. The following models will be presented: (1) collaborative practice, (2) professional nursing case management/relationship-based, (3) focused case management, and (4) two current working prototypes that will be called Model A and Model B. Using one of these models or pieces from each to blend into a unique model can be valuable to create a new or different CM role.

Collaborative Practice Model

The Collaborative Practice Model[4] (Figure 5-3) places the client at the apex of the pyramid, denoting their control in health care because the patient should be the driver on the path to wellness.

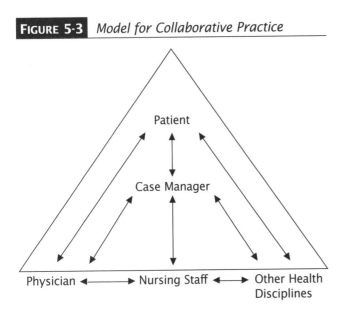

FIGURE 5-3 *Model for Collaborative Practice*

Reprinted with permission from Nugent, K. (1999). The clinical nurse specialist as case manager in a collaborative practice model: Bridging the gap between quality and cost of care. *Clinical Nurse Specialist, 6,* 106–111.

Dezell, Comeau, and Zander[15] state that patient care is integrated and comprehensive. This model is created through standards, CareMaps®, or clinical guidelines that drive the care process by a strict time line, directed by specific actions that result in predictable outcomes. These specific actions identify the interdisciplinary treatment plan, including any medications, procedures, therapies, and nursing care needed to restore the patient to a healthy condition. The collaborative practice model includes the following components: (1) forming a joint practice committee at the unit level, (2) instituting primary nursing as the model for delivery of patient care, (3) incorporating independent and interdependent decision making, (4) utilizing an integrated patient record, and (5) performing collaborative evaluation of patient care.[15]

For the Collaborative Practice Model to be successful, the CM needs to have a strong and very positive relationship with physicians and case managers throughout the organization. The plan should be established according to the nursing process, including assessment, analysis, implementation, and evaluation.[15] During the assessment process, patients and families are interviewed and data is gathered to formulate a needs assessment. After analyzing the assessment data, consider a guideline for care taking into account the barriers that would impede the expected outcomes.[15] This information is shared with the physician and primary nurse, and together the team would agree on a plan of care for the patient. The information is then documented on the patient's care path and shared with the team.[15] It is the responsibility of the CM to follow up on the patient, whether as an admission or a discharge.

Professional Nursing Case Management/Relationship-Based Model

Another model to consider is the Professional Nursing Case Management/Relationship-Based Model (PNCM) (Figure 5-4).[16] This model integrates nursing services across the care continuum, including community follow-up of the patient. The PNCM model provides the perfect opportunity to expand current working relationships with visiting nurses or home health nurses to develop a

- Establishing ongoing partnerships with clients
- Providing continuity as the client moves through the spectrum of health care settings
- Working with the client or family to seek the health care services at a lower severity of illness
- Integrating care during and beyond the acute episode of illness
- Facilitating timely access to health care resources and services
- Collaborating with primary nurses and other health care providers to promote cost-effective, quality care
- Promoting health maintenance and wellness
- Assisting clients to identify their options and understanding the consequences of their choices

community nurse health network. The essence of this model is relationship based. This model is unique because the relationships the CM forms with the patient, community, and health care community are integral to the success of the model. Relationships the patient has formed within their family, community, and personal network help to provide direction for the APN in planning care. This model calls for the APN to delve into the relationships of the patients and their families to come up with a plan that will provide the competent and cost-effective care the patient deserves. Interventions within the framework include (1) telling the story, (2) advancing the plan of care, (3) maintaining values and beliefs, and (4) assisting with options and decisions.[16]

The PNCM model introduces the "caring dimension" into the case management picture. It focuses on the ability of the CM to reach out and touch the patient and caregivers. Too often, the role of the CM is seen as cost driven and lacking in caring principles. Does this make us uncaring? Swanson has described five caring behaviors within the nurse–patient relationship. Reviewing these behaviors may be helpful for the CM when seeking ways to connect with patients and families. The five caring behaviors are (1) maintaining belief, (2) knowing, (3) being with, (4) doing for, and (5) enabling. She defines maintaining belief as sustaining faith in the other's capacity to get through an event or transition and face a future with meaning. Knowing is defined as striving to understand an event as it has meaning in the life of the other. Being with means being emotionally present for the other person. Doing for is doing for the other, as one would want done for oneself. Enabling is facilitating the other's safe passage through life transitions and unfamiliar events.[16]

This caring dimension should be built in as a quality indicator and included in the outcomes management report.

Focused Case Management Model

In addition to these two models, ED patients who are often seeking episodic care benefit from a Focused Case Management Model (FCM) (Figure 5-5). This model was developed by a Midwestern community-based ED and provides valuable insight of how to make case management work in an ED setting. The first step in putting the FCM model into practice is to identify the group of high-risk, high-cost patients to be managed. The CM consults with physicians, hospital administrators, finance officers, and statisticians to determine the group of patients to be managed. In the ED, the obvious group of patients most needing FCM would be the elderly, those with chronic illness, those noncompliant with medical regimes, and those with no insurance coverage. Other criteria used to select patients managed by the FCM model include (1) complex physiology (patients at high risk for complications or those requiring newer treatment modalities), (2) challenging family or ethical dynamics (staff nurses routinely assess family dynamics and request case management services when a family is in crisis and straining to make ethical decisions about the level of care), (3) fragmentation of care, possibly related to multiple medical providers or multiple caregivers,[17] (4) an anticipated length of stay that would be beyond current reimbursement that would put a financial burden on the family, (5) readmission less than 30 days after an inpatient discharge, and (6) primary care use of the emergency department for chronic illness.

FIGURE 5-5 *Focused Case Management Model*

Dashboard of Case Management-Sensitive Financial Indicators[6]

CEO/CFO		CNO/Director of Case Management	
Average cost per case	_____	Average cost per case	_____
Readmission rate <31 days postdischarge	_____	Readmission rate <31 days postdischarge	_____
Average length of stay versus industry standard	_____	Average length of stay versus industry standard	_____
Average cost per discharge	_____	Average length of stay (ICU and total acute care days)	_____
Admissions per 1,000	_____	Distribution of length of stay by patient population	_____
Patient days per 1,000	_____		
Admission frequency per DRG	_____	Physician satisfaction with case management services	_____
Total number of ED visits <31 days postdischarge	_____	Average change in SF-36 scores[7] (one year)	_____
		Case Management Productivity:	
		■ Average caseload per case manager	_____
		■ Hours per case	_____
		■ Contacts per month	_____
		■ Percentage of patients discharged with home health follow-up	_____

Differing Agendas

The preceding financial indicators provide a snapshot of the case management-sensitive data that hospital executives may use to evaluate the financial impact of case management services

Once the patient population to be managed is delineated, a plan of care is designed for a specific patient group. Criteria used to design the plan of care include (1) availability of family or caregivers to monitor care; (2) assistance in managing the interaction among primary, acute, transitional, or long-term care; (3) educational needs of health care workers, family, or caregivers to manage the illness more effectively; (4) availability of resources to provide needed equipment; and (5) a personal advocate to help manage within the health care system.[17]

The CM establishes the criteria for admission, transfer, and discharge based on ED and inpatient financial data; clinical outcome data; patient, physician, and staff satisfaction reports; home health and visiting nurse capabilities; and most frequent diagnosis/ICD-9 codes used in the emergency department. The CM leads process meetings to create guidelines for care, financial performa, integrated community resources, caring practices, and expected professional performance. Finally, the APN tracks progress through accurate and thoughtful record keeping, statistical measurements, satisfaction data and financial analysis.

Working Models

MODEL A

In Model A, CMs are assigned to a principal "at-risk" diagnosis-related group (DRG). Once the DRG is identified, the CM works within a team of health care professionals to develop guidelines for care and admission protocols for their specific DRG(s). The CM then educates the ED physicians and nurses, inpatient unit staff, and primary physicians on the care to be implemented. Outliers are discussed at monthly case management and utilization review meetings to evaluate patient outcomes and compliance with the guidelines and protocols.

The CM is then alerted to all potential admissions in her or his DRG group from the ED staff and responds to the ED to initiate an inquiry during daytime hours. Obviously, because the CM is devoted to a specific DRG group, she/he is not ED based. After hours, the CMs rotate call for admissions to ensure continuous attention to clinical guidelines and protocols. If the patient is admitted to the inpatient unit, the case manager who is responsible for a certain DRG(s) will then follow the patient through to discharge. Once discharged, the CMs work closely with the primary physician's office staff and any community agencies to ensure that the patient is compliant with the at-home plan of care. This continuum of care not only has had a marked decrease on inpatient recidivism, but also has decreased ED usage (Figure 5-6).

MODEL B

Model B is a computer-based model designed to track ED patients who are case managed from triage through discharge. This model is still in its infancy but looks very promising in terms of usability and efficiency. Once the computer identifies the patient entered as a "case-managed" patient, the patient care guidelines and protocols identified by the CM are displayed on the screen so all health care professionals caring for the patient are made aware of the recommendations. Model B also has the potential to alert ED staff when a patient is a chronic ED user as to the care guidelines that were agreed on by the emergency physicians and patient (as well as the primary care physician/consultant, if applicable). This model looks promising for improved screenings, and referrals to community agencies and decreasing health care utilization costs.

In addition to the models discussed, there are other models that integrate utilization review, social service, and case management all into one role; still, there are others that separate two or three of the roles. There are no standard models that work for every ED; however, the concepts and constructs of all models are similar. The best advice is to conduct a thorough assessment based on individual ED data to determine the most appropriate model.

Summary

The role of the CM is intense. The CM is responsive to administrative concerns as well as concerns from patients, staff, and community agencies. Will CMs be ready to answer the call in the name of professional nurses everywhere? CMs set the stage for the future of nursing, leading health care into a transformation that responds to the call of those in need of wellness. Success for the role has been varied due to lack of clarity and defensiveness from those in utilization review positions, social service, and physicians who misunderstand and see their practices being challenged.[16] Lack of planning, expertise, and authority, as well as differing agendas, have also been instrumental in loosing leverage on case management.

Because of rising ED volumes, diminished health care resources, and reduced health care dollars, there is a need for CMs to meet the unfilled medical needs of patients and families. As technology offers more alternatives to life, the population ages, and the aging have more life, it is essential for hospitals to provide much-needed care to the patients by the one professional who has always been there for patients, 24 hours a day. Professional services are provided by the one health care worker who has respect, advanced education, experience, compassion, and trustworthiness. Who better to fill the role than the CM?

REFERENCES

1. Flaherty, L. (2002). Visits to the emergency department increase. *Journal of Emergency Nursing, 28*(5), 447–448.
2. Centers for Disease Control. (2002). Visits to the emergency department increase nationwide. National hospital ambulatory medical care survey: 2000. *Emergency department summary.* Washington, DC: National Center for Health Statistics. U.S. Department of Health and Human Services.
3. Given, B. A. (2001). Nurse practitioners: Issues within a managed care environment. In J. M. Dochterman & H. K. Grace (Eds.), *Current issues in nursing* (6th ed., pp. 358–365). St. Louis, MO: Mosby.
4. Nugent, K. (1999). The clinical nurse specialist as case manager in a collaborative practice model: Bridging the gap between quality and cost of care. *Clinical Nurse Specialist, 6*(2), 106–111.

FIGURE 5-6 *Model A: Algorithm for Patient Placement*

Emergency Department Case Management Algorithm

		↓	
	Evaluated by Triage RN		
↙		↘	
Does not meet case management criteria		Meets Case management criteria	
↓		↓	
Seen by ED physician		APRN interviews patient/caregivers	
		↓	
		APRN performs ROS assessment	
		↓	
		APRN collaborates with ED physician and nurse	
		↓	
		Action plan implemented for clinical guidelines and management plan	
		↓	
	Patient disposition		
↙	↓		↘
Discharge home	To be admitted		Home with community help
↓	↙	↘	↓
Family available to assist	Meets criteria	Does not meet criteria	APRN contacts relative, community services to implement action plan for care at home.
↓	↙	↘	↓
APRN and primary care nurse provide written and verbal educational materials to patient and family	Admitting physician is contacted for orders; patient is admitted to nursing unit with guidelines for care	Alternatives for noninpatient care are explored and an outpatient care plan is implemented with the community team	APRN and community team meet to review care plan with patient
Return communication is demonstrated from patient and family	APRN turns case management over to inpatient case		
Follow appt. (48 hrs) is made with Primary physician	Upon discharge, if patient is in need of continuous care, the record will show "case managed" to alert all caregivers of plan		↗
APRN contacts patient within 24 hrs. Patient is: Better—keep appt. Same—keep appt. Worse—Patient/family/APRN contact physician for direction/orders			

APRN—Advanced practice registered nurse; ROS—review of systems.

5. Leberman, A., & Rotarius, T. (1999). Managed care evolution: Where did it come from and where is it going? In C. Eleanor (Ed.), *Nursing issues in the 21st century: Perspectives from the literature* (pp. 423–431). Philadelphia: Lippincott, Williams & Wilkins.

6. Elixhauser, A., Yu, K., Steiner, C., & Bierman, A. S. (2000). Hospitalization in the United States, 1997 (HCUP Fact book No. 1, AHRQ Publication No. 00-0031). Rockville, MD: Agency for Healthcare Resource and Quality.

7. Harrison, J. (2001). Influence of managed care on professional nursing practice. *Image: Journal of Nursing Scholarship, 32*(2), 161–166.

8. American Nurses Association. (1996). *Scope and standards of advanced practice registered nursing.* Washington, DC: Author.

9. Nursing Executive Center—Healthcare Advisory Board. (1999). *Prioritization of target populations for care management and process improvement activities.* Washington, DC: Advisory Board Company.

10. del Bueno, D. J., Griffin, L. R., Burke, S. M., & Foley, M. A. (1990). The clinical teacher: A critical link to competence development. *Journal of Nursing Staff Development, 6*(3), 135–138.

11. Porter-O'Grady, T., & Krueger Wilson, C. (1996). *The leadership revolution in health care: Altering systems, changing behaviors.* Gaithersburg, MD: Aspen.

12. Sandrick, K. (1994). Managing managed care. Corporate network managers have a portfolio of new responsibilities. *Hospitals and Health Networks, 68*(20), 58, 60, 62.

13. Witbeck, G., Hornfield, S., & Dalack, G. W. (2000). Emergency room outreach to chronically addicted individuals: A pilot study. *Journal of Substance Abuse, 19*(1), 39–43.

14. Flarey, D. L., & Blancett, S. S. (1996). Health care delivery in a world of managed care. *The Journal of Care Management, 2*(3), 22–34.

15. Dezell, A. V., Comeau, E., & Zander, K. (1987). Nursing case management: Managed care via the nursing case management model. *NLN Publications, 20,* 253–264.

16. Sohl-Kreiger, R., Lagaard, M. W., & Scherrer, J. (1996). Nursing case management: Relationship as a strategy to improve care. *Clinical Nurse Specialist, 10*(2), 107–109.

17. Brewer, B. B., & Jackson, L. (1997). A case management model for the emergency department. *Journal of Emergency Nursing, 23*(6), 618–621.

6 INFORMATICS IN THE EMERGENCY DEPARTMENT

Mary Hardesty, RN, FNP, MS

Introduction

Information technology has become an integral part of patient care and is essential knowledge for advanced practice nurses (APNs) practicing in today's emergency departments (ED). Informatics is the study and application of computer and statistical techniques for the management of information. Information overload is a common complaint of health care professionals. What information is the most current and most reliable? Where can I get the most up-to-date information regarding my ED practice? Society and medicine are changing rapidly; health care providers are challenged to become proficient in the ability to both access and critique current information. Effectively integrating information technology with the care of patients is vital to how we manage patients and improve care in emergency medicine. This chapter will discuss the importance of information technology to the practice of APNs in the ED and guide the APN regarding current and future directions in information technology.

Medical informatics is defined as the use of information technology, communication tools, and computer systems to enhance and improve all aspects of patient care, medical education, and medical research.[1] Medical informatics is also used by health care workers to advance and teach knowledge about the application of information and technologies to health care—the place in which health information and computer sciences, psychology, epidemiology, and engineering intersect.[2] Thus informatics combine computer science and information science to process data and information. Information is collected, organized, analyzed, managed, and then used in health care. Medical informatics incorporates the skills of gathering, analyzing, managing, and using information in health care.[3,4]

Increased usage of computers by the public, specifically health care professionals and patients, has provided information to medical personnel, enhancing delivery of patient care. The APN can use this knowledge of informatics to search the Internet, correspond via e-mail, participate in interactive forums, use telemedicine technology, search databases, and conduct research.

Internet

The Internet is a computerized source of information that provides the computer user with rapid information on a variety of topics and facilitates the exchange of ideas instantly. Today much information about medicine, technology, and patient care is available via the Internet. Over 98 million people in the United States use the Internet as a source of medical information.[5] Patients can also gather medical information using the Internet to collaborate with health care providers, becoming part of the decision-making process. APNs that have working knowledge of the Internet not only enhance their own knowledge but also help patients comprehend the information they find.

General Information

The growth of the Internet is overwhelming. A little over 40 years ago, when computers were in their infancy, four computers comprised the state-of-the-art computer network. By 1985 there were over 600 computers in the United States, and currently over 50 million people use computers.[6]

Getting connected to the Internet is accomplished by either slow- or high-speed connectors. The connection is accessed through a telephone modem, cable modem, or digital subscriber lines (DSL). Slow speed is accomplished via dial-up access by a telephone modem that send signals over phone lines with varying speed. Cable modems provide high-speed connections to the Internet from a local cable provider whereas DSLs carry information over telephone wires via bandwidth or frequency at a speed three to four times faster than a modem. Slow-speed modem is available to anyone with a telephone. The speed at which information is transmitted is slower, and clarity with video is not as clear as with high-speed access.

Once the access mode is determined, the Internet is available to anyone. The Internet comprises different individual components. The "www" is an abbreviation for World Wide Web and appears in Web addresses. The www can transmit text, graphics, and other media rapidly using browsers. A Web browser is a software program that is used to view pages on the Web. Microsoft Internet Explorer® and Netscape® are examples of software programs that carry Internet information. To get to a page on the www, you have to know the address of the Web page, or URL (uniform resource locator). Sending Web pages to a browser occurs through hypertext transfer protocol, http://. Web addresses start with this text to let the browser know to be ready to display the Web page. Web pages are developed using Hypertext Markup Language (HTML), which is a series of tags or codes that are embedded in a document to describe how the page should look when viewed by a browser.

More definitions for computer-related lingo are available on the following Web site: http://webopedia.internet.com.

WEB PAGES

Web pages contain information that sells products or services or gives information. They are constructed for a variety of reasons. For example, they provide access to news, entertainment, culture, travel, health, and wellness. Through a Web page, a person can share information and contribute to the Web.

ACCESS

Internet service providers (ISPs) are independent companies that provide access to the Internet.

ISPs, such as CompuServe and AOL, provide news, e-mail, discussion groups, files for downloading, and other online services to subscribers. Organizational providers such as local colleges or universities, health care agencies, governmental agencies, or libraries are available and offer limited free usage of the Internet.[7]

Purposes

Because the Internet is available 24 hours a day, information can be gathered at one's convenience. Through the Internet, an abundance of information and resources is available to health care professionals such as medical information, including patient education and research, newsgroups, libraries, e-journals, and medical books.

Communication Systems

E-MAIL

E-mail is the most commonly used service on the Internet today. One keystroke can send a communication to a person in the next town, state, country, or continent in a few seconds.[8] Many APNs are now using e-mail as a way to communicate with patients, families, and other health care workers.

Using the Internet to facilitate communication between health care workers and their patients has come under much scrutiny because of legal, ethical, and privacy issues. E-mail can be easily altered, forwarded, or duplicated. Identity verification, technology failure, timeliness of responses, and confidentiality are other considerations that affect the health care provider when using e-mail in practice.[1]

Another concern for the health care provider is the lack of computer access by all patients. Many patients either cannot afford a computer or lack the knowledge and expertise necessary to navigate the Internet.

Although e-mail can enhance and promote patient well-being by communicating educational materials, instructions, appointment reminders, or prescription refills, it does not have the availability to reach all patients, whereas the phone and regular mail has proven useful for this purpose in the past.[8]

LISTSERVS

A listserv is a computer program that allows a number of people with similar interests to communicate with each other via e-mail. The program maintains a list of the group's e-mail addresses and acts as an e-mail message distributor for its members.[9]

Telemedicine

Telemedicine uses communication technology to exchange health-related information over a distance for patient care. The telephone was the first technology used. Now health care providers can transmit radiographs, medical records, and lab results to online consultants through connections such as DSL, modems, or dedicated Internet lines.[10] Health care lectures, seminars, even surgeries can be transmitted via telemedicine. Telemedicine is an invaluable tool when information needs to be broadcasted to a large number of health care workers across the nation.

Clinical Decision Support Systems

Technological advances such as the Internet have brought information to the health care provider in the clinical environment. Clinical decision support systems provide a common standardized structure for the electronic medical record and a type of tracking service for specific information, such as outcome and performance indicators. One example of a clinical decision support system is a computerized decision support (CDS) system. A CDS system is a medical knowledge base server that can assist with diagnosis and management of illness and improve patient care. These systems can also provide preventative care components specific for each patient.[11]

When time is of the utmost importance, locating reliable information becomes vital. Many databases are available that provide information and guidelines for emergency health care providers. Several of these databases are listed in Table 6-1.

SEARCH ENGINES

Performing a search involves using a search engine, which searches a database to match contents in the database to the question. Search engines differ in user friendliness and their ability to perform complicated searches. Some examples of search engines are google.com, yahoo.com, and altavista.com.

Information Systems

Information systems in health care include clinical, financial, social, and research data and are used to track epidemiological surveys as well as specific health care information, health care costs, and research. This information is used to defend current practice, suggest best-practice models and predict future health care needs and goals.

Medical Record

Historically, the medical record was developed to store information and to communicate among personnel to provide continuity and documentation of care. Medical records were often handwritten, and data were manually entered. Problems with the written medical record included (1) time involved in finding the record, (2) poor organization, (3) poor legibility, and (4) lost records. Currently, it is estimated that over $90 billion is wasted each year because medical histories are not available to health care providers.

The electronic medical record (EMR) is quickly replacing the standard medical record. The EMR encompasses processes that were once performed manually and can now link diagnoses to billing, quality control measures, patient tracking records, and legal and finance reference.[6] Electronic information systems provide ease with record retrieval, are legible, and can be accessed by several individuals at one time. The EMR can provide reminders or alerts, can perform calculations, and is always available.[12]

However, the EMR is not without problems: (1) the system is costly, (2) personnel must be trained to use the system, (3) security concerns are high, (4) data entry can be difficult, and (4) technology can fail. Maintaining a secure environment within the electronic medical record becomes of utmost importance so that sensitive patient information is not compromised.

Table 6-1

Databases	
DATABASE	CHARACTERISTICS
MEDLINE	■ Large bibliographic database maintained by U.S. National Library of Medicine[13] ■ Consists of more than 3,900 current biomedical journals ■ Can be accessed through two free access engines: PubMed: http://www.ncbi.nlm.nih.gov/entrez/query.fcgi National Library of Medicine Gateway: http://www.gateway.nlm.nih.gov/gw/Cmd[14]
Cochrane Library	■ Contains the collected work of the Cochrane Collaboration, an international organization that prepares, maintains, and disseminates systematic reviews of randomized trials of health care interventions ■ Clinical problems are addressed using a meta-analysis of all research on the clinical problems. The research is analyzed and suggestions for practice are recommended. ■ Access: http://www.cochrane.org
American College of Physicians (ACP) Journal Club	■ Contains summaries of studies, abstracts, and article reviews from 125 journals from 1991 to the present ■ Access: http://www.acpjc.org
National Center for Emergency Medicine Informatics (NCEMI)	■ Comprehensive online library of emergency medicine informatics ■ Provides tools and information for medical informatics searches, Medline searches, software for ED, and hot links to medical sites, including clinical tools, textbook references, practice guidelines, and many other resources ■ Included in this site is JADE (journal abstracts delivered electronically), which searches MEDLINE each week on a customized search requested by e-mail ■ Access: http://www.ncemi.org
American Nurses Association (ANA)	■ Professional national organization for RNs throughout the U.S. ■ Access: www.nursingworld.org
World Health Organization (WHO)	■ Specialized agency for health with the objective of the attainment of the highest level of health by all people ■ Includes links to reports, information sources, etc. ■ Access: www.who.int/en
National Institutes of Health (NIH)	■ A link to the U.S. Department of Health and Human Services that provides health information such as publications and fact sheets, clinical trials, health hotlines, health topics from A–Z, and more ■ Access: www.nih.gov
National Institute Nursing Research (NINR)	■ A link to the NIH and provides a clinical and nursing perspective to biomedical and behavioral research ■ Access: www.nih.gov/ninr/
American College of Nurse Practitioners (ACNP)	■ National nonprofit membership organization for nurse practitioners (NPs) ■ Keeps NPs current on political and professional issues ■ Access: www.nurse.org/acnp/
NP Central	■ Provides information for NPs, including continuing education listings, NP programs, job listings, and classes for enhancing NP practice ■ Offers listservs for discussion among member NPs ■ Access: www.npcentral.net

Personal Digital Assistants

Personal digital assistants (PDAs) have revolutionized health care. A PDA is a small, handheld minicomputer that keeps track of appointments, stores phone numbers, handles wireless e-mail and messaging, stores clinical information, takes digital photographs, and can even provide a cellular phone service.

Software programs are available for PDAs that provide up-to-date medical tools to enhance patient care. These programs can be accessed and downloaded from the Internet. Some clinical software such as ePocrates Rx™, Tarascon Pocket Pharmacopoeia™, (drug information), and Preg-Calc can be obtained free of charge. Other databases are available for a fee, such as The 5-Minute Clinical Consult, and PEPID™, an emergency medicine palm-based text. Table 6-2 lists several texts that can be downloaded to a PDA and various Websites that provide access to additional software programs.

Research

Research remains essential to health care and a significant component of the APN role. Informatics can help present research findings at the point of care to influence practice behavior. Data can be collected, stored, analyzed, displayed, and integrated. Through the integration of data from one or more information sources, information can be linked together. This links researchers through networking and improves research findings.[15] Single EDs can join collaborative research networks establishing a large database for research. In this regard, the computer age has changed clinical practice significantly.

Summary

Health care is changing rapidly in large part because of the lightning-speed progression of information technology. Health care providers must become proficient with the use of information technology. Quick access to relevant and valid data of all types is imperative. Improved information management by all health care providers will enhance and advance patient care and assist with

research in the future. Using the computer to document findings and connect patient care to billing and cost of services can only enhance the practice of the APN. Not only can the Internet provide the APN with valuable resources to improve communication with patients, families, and other health care providers, but it can also put the information and knowledge of the world's leading experts in the pocket of the APN.

Table 6-2

PDA Clinical Software

PDA Textbooks:
  Merck Manual: Centennial Edition
  Taber's Cyclopedic Medical Dictionary
  DSM-IV: Text Revision
  Nursing Care Plans
  Harrison's Principles of Internal Medicine
  Principles of Critical Care
  Washington Mnl™ (The Washington Manual of Medical Therapeutics)
  5-Minute Emergency Medicine Consult
  Advanced Cardiac Life Support 2000
  PEPID™

Pharmacopedics
  ePocrates (www.epocrates.com)
  Lexi-Drugs™ (www.lexi.com)
  Physicians' Desk Reference® (www.pdr.net)
  Physician's Drug Handbook (www.handheldmed.com)
  Tarascon Pocket Pharmacopoeia (www.tarasconpublishing.com)

PDA Websites:
  http://avantgo.com
  http://www.collectivemed.com
  http://www.epocrates.com
  http://www.eurocool.com
  http://www.freewarepalm.com
  http://www.handango.com
  http://www.handheldmed.com
  http://www.healthypalmpilot.com
  http://www.lexi.com
  http://www.medicalpiloteer.com
  http://www.medscape.com
  http://www.palmgear.com
  http://www.palmpilotarchives.com
  http://www.patientkeeper.com
  http://www.pdacortex.com
  http://www.pdamd.com
  http://www.pdr.net
  http://www.pilotzone.com
  http://www.skyscape.com
  http://www.softwarenirvana.com
  http://www.tucows.com

REFERENCES

1. Kulkarni, R., & Nathanson, L. A. (2001). Medical informatics in emergency medicine. Retrieved November 20, 2002 from http://www.emedicine.com/emerg/topic879.htm

2. What is medical informatics—some formal definitions of the field. (n.d.). Retrieved November 20, 2002 from http://www.amia.org/search/fsearch.html

3. Graves, J. R., & Corcoran, S. (1989). The study of nursing informatics. *Image: Journal of Nursing Scholarship, 21*(4), 227–231.

4. Barnett, O. (1990). Computers in medicine. *JAMA, 263*(19), 2631–2633.

5. Rajendran, P. (2001). Using the Internet: Ushering in a new era of medicine. Retrieved November 20, 2002 from http://www.ama-assn.org/sci-pubs/msjama/articles/vol_285/no_5/jms0214011.htm

6. Cordell, W., Overhage, J., & Waeckerle, J. (1998). Strategies for improving information management in emergency medicine to meet clinical, research, and administrative needs. *Annals of Emergency Medicine, 5*(2), 162–167.

7. Feied, C., & Smith, M. (1996). An emergency medicine physician lost in the Internet. Retrieved November 20, 2002 from http://www.ncemi.org/eddocuments/1a-inet2.htm

8. Kane, B., & Sands, D. Z. (1998). Guidelines for the clinical use of electronic mail with patients. The AMIA Internet working group, task force on guidelines for the use of clinic-patient electronic mail. *Journal of the American Medical Informatics Association, 5*(1), 104–111.

9. What is a listserv? (n.d.). Retrieved November 20, 2002 from http://www.aanp.org/whatisalistserv.htm

10. Wootton, R. (2001). Recent advances: Telemedicine. *British Medical Journal, 323*(7312), 557–560.

11. Coiera, R. (1997). Introduction to medical informatics. In *Guide to medical informatics, the Internet, and telemedicine.* [Electronic version]. Retrieved November 20, 2002 from http://www.coiera.com/bk-intro.htm

12. Teich, J. M. (1998). Information systems support for emergency medicine. *Annals of Emergency Medicine, 5*(3), 271–274.

13. Corrall, C. J., Wyer, P. C., Zick, L. S., & Bockrath, C. R. (2002). Evidence-based emergency medicine. How to find evidence when you need it, part 1: Databases, search programs, and strategies. *Annals of Emergency Medicine, 39*(3), 302–306.

14. Gallagher, P. E., Allen, T. Y., & Wyer, P. C. (2002). How to find evidence when you need it, part 3: A clinician's guide to MEDLINE: Tricks and special skills. *Annals of Emergency Medicine, 39*(5), 547–551.

PART THREE

ADVANCED PRACTICE

7

THE ROLE OF THE CLINICAL NURSE SPECIALIST IN THE EMERGENCY DEPARTMENT

Jean A. Proehl, RN, MN, CEN, CCRN

What Is a Clinical Nurse Specialist?

Definition

Clinical nurse specialists (CNSs) are advanced practice nurses (APNs) who are expert clinicians and client advocates in a specific specialty or subspecialty of nursing.[1] Master's or doctoral education including supervised clinical practice is a prerequisite to advanced practice nursing,[1,2] and in addition, an APN has "ongoing clinical experiences."[1]

Regulatory Requirements

Regulatory and licensing requirements vary widely from state to state, and in many instances, the title "Clinical Nurse Specialist" is used by virtue of the institutional role one is hired to fill. However, many states now specifically authorize CNS services and require that the CNS receive formal recognition from the state board of nursing as a CNS; some states even require a second license. Prerequisites for a state's recognition of a CNS vary. All states that formally recognize CNS practice require a master's degree, and almost all specify that it must be from a program that prepares CNS graduates.[3] Some states require certification as a CNS or may accept certification in the specialty area of nursing if no specialty CNS exam is available. Currently, there is no certification examination for emergency CNSs.

Eight states do not formally recognize CNSs, and 7 states limit CNS recognition to psychiatric–mental health CNSs.[3] Only 20 states have a distinct CNS scope of practice; 21 states have identical licensing and scope of practice requirements for CNSs and nurse practitioners (NPs).[3] These licensing or recognition requirements are very im-portant for CNSs seeking direct reimbursement, independent practice involving direct care of patients, or prescriptive authority.

Role

"What is a CNS?" and "What does a CNS do?" are probably the most common questions all CNSs are asked about their job. Nurses, physicians, other health care providers, and laypeople alike are often unfamiliar with the role.[4] Because the role is multifaceted and flexible, it may be easier to explain what the role does *not* encompass than what it does encompass. The CNS role does not usually include administrative functions such as hiring, firing, staffing and scheduling, disciplinary action, or budgeting. However, even though CNSs may not have the authority or responsibility for those processes, they should have some input into these functions as they pertain to clinical care.

Simply put, a CNS promotes and provides support for safe and effective patient care. This support involves activities within three spheres of influence: patient/family, nurse–nurse, and system. In each of these spheres, eight interventions are seen as essential to the CNS role: (1) clinical judgment, (2) clinical inquiry, (3) facilitation of learning, (4) collaboration, (5) systems thinking, (6) advocacy/moral agency, (7) caring practices, and (8) response to diversity (see Table 7-1).[5]

Components of the Role

The traditional components of the CNS role include expert clinical practice, education, research, leadership, and consultation. A sample job description encompassing these traditional role components is found in Appendix A. The activities of a specific CNS are dependent on the practice

Table 7-1

Clinical Nurse Specialist Interventions in the Three Spheres of Influence

NURSE DIMENSION	PATIENT/FAMILY	NURSE–NURSE	SYSTEM
Clinical judgment	Synthesize, interpret, and make decisions based on complex, sometimes conflicting, sources of data	Facilitate development of clinical judgment in health care team members (e.g., nursing staff, medical staff, other health care providers) through role modeling, teaching, coaching, and/or mentoring	Develop, implement and evaluate research-based algorithms, decision trees, protocols, and care plans for patients and patient populations
Clinical inquiry	Using research-based evidence/outcome data, formulate, evaluate, and/or revise policies, procedures, protocols, individualized patient care programs, and standards for care	Role model, teach, coach, and/or mentor nursing staff regarding the use and evaluation of research findings	Drawing on resources including the literature, benchmarking studies, and colleagues, design and evaluate innovations in clinical practice affecting patients/populations and/or systems
Facilitator of learning	Collaborate with patient/family, nursing staff, medical staff, and other health care professionals to develop, implement, and evaluate education programs based on learner needs	Facilitate nursing staff development of patient education-related skills (e.g., needs assessment, evaluation of learner understanding, integrating education throughout delivery of care)	Contribute to and advance the knowledge base of the health care community through presentations, publications, and involvement in professional organizations
Collaboration	Lead or participate in multidisciplinary teams to develop programs based on patient care issues	Role model, teach, coach, and/or mentor professional leadership and accountability for nursing's role within the health care team	Involve/recruit diverse resources to optimize patient outcomes
Systems thinking	Develop, integrate, apply, and evaluate a variety of strategies that are driven by the needs and strengths of the patients/family, nursing staff, medical staff, and other health care professionals	Role model, teach, coach, and/or mentor creative/innovative systems thinking and resources use among nursing staff	Integrate knowledge of organizational mission, goals, and systems into patient care strategy, development, and implementation. Anticipate possible consequences of systems change, and develop proactive strategies.
Advocacy/moral agency	Establish an environment that promotes ethical decision making and patient advocacy	Facilitate development of nurse's advocacy and moral agency through role modeling, teaching, coaching, and mentoring	Develop community education programs in regard to such issues as living wills, advance directives, power of attorney, and organ donation
Caring practices	Develop and/or implement a process to ensure that patient/family needs are met in regard to body image, loss, healing, death, and dying/powerlessness	Facilitate development of nurses' caring practices through role modeling, teaching, coaching, and/or mentoring	Provide patient/family skills to navigate transitions along the health care continuum (e.g., facilitate safe passage)
Response to diversity	Recognize and integrate individual differences and complementary therapies into patient/family care	Identify issues arising from individual differences and develop awareness of these issues in nursing staff, medical staff, and other health care providers	Tailor the delivery of care, to the extent possible, to meet the diverse needs and strengths of patient/family, staff, and system

Reprinted with permission from Moloney-Harmon, P. A. (1999). The synergy model: Contemporary practice of the clinical nurse specialist. *Critical Care Nurse, 19*(2), 102.

environment, the needs of nursing staff and patients, and organizational expectations. Day-to-day activities often vary significantly as the CNS performs various components of the role.

One essential function in all subroles is information brokering. Deciding *what* information needs to be shared with *whom* along with *how* and *when* to share it are essential in today's Information Age. For example, when a memo comes from the pharmacy that a new medication has been added to the formulary, the CNS must first decide if it is likely that the medication will be used in the emergency department (ED). If the answer is yes, the CNS must investigate the nursing implications of procuring, storing, and administering the medication. Next, a mechanism for sharing the necessary information must be determined (e.g., e-mail, memo, classes, videotape, Web- or computer-based learning activity, or self-instructional module). In addition to initial education about the medication, the CNS must ensure that appropriate resources are present in the ED for future reference. This may be as simple as confirming that the information is in a standard medication reference available in the ED or as complex as developing a reference sheet with pharmacy and physician input. The CNS may also need to ensure that emergency physicians have received information about the medication and its potential impact on nursing and patient care.

A study looking at CNS roles and activities surveyed 724 practicing CNSs and found the following ranges for percentage of time spent in various components of the role: clinical practice 29% to 91%, education 24% to 89%, research 15% to 93%, leadership/administrative 34% to 85%, and consultation 18% to 96%.[6] These findings illustrate how much the role may vary in different settings.

Expert Clinical Practice

The clinical expertise component of the role is the cornerstone of CNS practice, and direct patient care is only one way in which CNSs are clinically active. Involvement in clinical practice occurs in a variety of ways, including coaching or assisting other nurses delivering direct patient care and introducing new clinical information or technology

for direct patient care. For patients with complex needs such as trauma or cardiac resuscitation, the CNS may be part of the team providing direct care. Helping out in times of high census/high acuity, troubleshooting equipment, and assisting nurses to resolve problematic patient care situations are other examples of CNS clinical practice. In some cases, CNSs coordinate clinics for special patient populations or perform medical procedures such as suturing, chest tube insertion, central line insertion, and intubation.[6] The APN that would typically perform advanced procedures is an emergency nurse practitioner, but a CNS with specific training, demonstrated competency, and institutional support may also function in this capacity if so permitted by the state's nurse practice act.

Education

Support for patient care via education is an important role component. Education may involve teaching in formal classes or conferences or it may be informal one-on-one teaching at the bedside. Information brokering, as described earlier, is an essential component of this subrole. CNSs teach nurses, physicians, other health care providers, students in various health care programs, patients, families, and communities (e.g., injury prevention and health promotion activities). Also included in the education role component is coordinating orientation for new employees and evaluating staff competency.

Research

CNS functions in the research role are not limited to actually conducting research; CNSs are in an ideal position to help bridge the gap between research and practice. Using research findings in practice, disseminating research findings, participating in product evaluation, assisting or collaborating with others to conduct research, writing grant proposals, participating in research committees and institutional review boards, and presenting research findings at seminars and conferences are all examples of the implementation of the research subrole. Many activities that fall under the guise of quality improvement involve research. For example, conducting interrater reliability studies of triage categorization and evaluating the impact of patient-controlled analgesia in ED patients with chest pain are examples of research activities that are also quality improvement activities.

Leadership

Leadership functions of CNSs involve informal and formal leadership. Many of the functions included in the subrole are administrative in nature. Some examples of leadership functions performed by CNSs include performing or providing input into performance appraisals or disciplinary actions, establishing and implementing goals related to nursing practice or patient care, providing input into the budgetary process or developing budgets, developing new programs, and supervising employees, including hiring, interviewing, and counseling. Leadership also encompasses involvement with institutional committees, shared governance, quality improvement, patient billing, and patient satisfaction activities. Specific examples for the emergency CNS include leading the nursing staff in the development of an ED-specific standard of care or the implementation of a new triage system.

Consultation

Providing clinical consultation to nurses in other specialty areas is a part of every CNS's role and is a major role component for population-based CNSs. Consultation activities are diverse and include developing and implementing policies and procedures, serving on organizational task forces and committees, collaborating with leadership to identify and solve problems, facilitating support groups, and serving on editorial or grant review boards. Emergency CNSs are frequently asked to consult in the development of systems and plans for emergency situations in nonemergency or critical care areas (e.g., cardiac arrest or sudden patient deterioration on a medical-surgical unit). Participating in organizational task forces and committees addressing sedation, restraint, blood administration, trauma care, and medication administration are other common consultative activities for emergency CNSs.

Nontraditional Subroles

In addition to the traditional role components described earlier, CNSs have found that their knowledge and skill set are transferable to other roles.

CASE MANAGEMENT

Case management typically focuses on high-risk and high-cost patient populations. It encompasses direct patient care, financial management, prevention, patient education, and analysis of outcomes. Continuity of care delivered in a cost-effective manner is a key goal of case management and is congruent with the goals of the traditional CNS role. Formal CNS educational preparation may not include case management principles, and so other methods of attaining this knowledge base may be necessary. However, some argue that CNSs are overqualified for this role, and it would be better to use their expertise and research background to supervise case managers (CMs) instead of functioning as CMs.[7] In fact, a BSN, not graduate education, is often required for some CM position. CMs (not necessarily CNSs) are employed in many EDs, and some ED CNSs have a case management component to their role. In the ED, case management frequently focuses on patients and populations that are heavy users of emergency services. For example, patients with poorly controlled chronic diseases such as sickle cell anemia, asthma, or diabetes tend to visit the ED frequently and may benefit from a coordinated and consistent approach to their care.

ORGANIZATION DEVELOPMENT

CNSs may be used in place of outside consultants in an organization development capacity. The focus of the role becomes improvement of systems and organizational culture. This model can provide a cost-effective internal consultant who already has established alliances with the nursing and medical staffs and who is an experienced change agent. An added advantage is that the CNS is a permanent employee who is available for follow-up work as needed.[8] Spearheading the development and implementation of a standard sedation policy and procedure throughout the organization is one example of how an ED CNS might serve in an organization development capacity. Sedation is performed in many different areas, and implementation of a standard policy and procedure requires the involvement and buy-in of a wide variety of people and departments, from anesthesiology to audiology and many places in between. The changes necessary to implement a standard sedation procedure may require a shift in organizational culture toward patient safety in addition to new equipment, knowledge, and skills.

HOUSE STAFF REPLACEMENT

CNSs and NPs have been used to replace house staff as residency positions decreased and the needs of hospitalized patients became more complex. Some would argue that APNs are actually better qualified than house staff because of their commitment to the ED, knowledge of the system and policies/procedures, and expertise in patient management and nursing care principles. Traditional NP educational preparation is better suited to this subrole, but inherent in CNS practice is clinical expertise, which is required for this function. Some additional educational preparation may be required for the CNS to perform functions traditionally viewed as the responsibility of house staff. Licensing, reimbursement, credentialing, and privileging issues also need to be addressed. This subrole of CNS practice is rare in ED settings because emergency NPs are usually employed to meet these needs.

UNSPOKEN SUBROLES

No matter what the CNS job description includes with regard to the traditional subroles, there are always inherent, unspoken subroles. McCaffrey[9] uses analogies to describe the essence of how CNS subroles are accomplished (Table 7-2).

Actualization of the Role

Reporting Relationships

Most CNSs report to a senior administrator such as an assistant vice president, director of a specialty area, vice president of nursing, or the chief nursing officer.[6] These senior administrators may or may not be nurses. However, in one study, 22% of CNSs reported to unit managers or physicians.[6] This may result in conflict because of dif-

Table 7-2	
The Unspoken Subroles of CNS Practice	
Detective	A collaborative problem-solving effort using expert knowledge and critical-thinking skills
Architect	Planning and building/remodeling projects and programs using coordinated input from others
Car salesman	Persuading others to buy their idea using informal power, influence, and motivational skills
Choreographer	Assist others to learn to do things in new ways
Mail carrier	Delivering news, both good and bad
Cheerleader	Giving positive feedback and encouragement
Priest	Confidant
Spring trainer	Collaborates in team development and team building
Crop duster	Disseminating information to key individuals to help navigate a change
Senator	Advocating for patients, families, nurses, other health care professionals, and the institution
Weatherman	Look to the future to predict changes in care delivery

Adapted with permission from McCaffrey, D. (1991). The unspoken subroles of the clinical nurse specialist. *Clinical Nurse Specialist, 5*(2), 71–72.

ferent role expectations. Collaboration with the unit manager is necessary to improve patient care and nursing practice, and a direct reporting relationship may make that difficult. Physicians tend to focus on the direct patient care aspects of the role and may not value other components.

CNSs may be in staff or line management positions. The advantages of a line management position include the authority to enforce clinical practice standards. A major disadvantage is that it places the CNS in a "boss" relationship, and this may make it difficult for nurses to confide in the CNS regarding self-perceived clinical inadequacies. The other responsibilities that come with line management also compete for the CNS's time and may overshadow the clinical role.[6]

Unit-Based versus Population-Based CNSs

Most emergency CNSs are unit based; that is, they are specifically assigned to the ED. Population-based CNSs may augment the role of unit-based CNSs by addressing specific patient populations. For example, psychiatric liaison, diabetes, trauma, and wound/ostomy are all example of population-based CNS practices that will intersect with emergency CNSs.

Role Barriers and Enhancers

Role confusion and differing perspectives on what the CNS's priorities should be can lead to dissatisfaction among the stakeholders. A collaborative relationship with nursing and physician leadership is essential to negotiate roles and responsibilities. It is important that these leaders then support the CNS's role with staff. Sponsorship by key individuals in nursing leadership has been cited as an important factor in CNS longevity.[10] Another barrier may be staff nurses' respect for and acceptance of the CNS as an expert clinician. CNSs usually need to demonstrate their clinical expertise on a regular (or at least frequent) basis to maintain credibility with the staff.

As recognition of CNSs' abilities and expertise spread, it is very easy for them to become overextended. There is almost no aspect of health care that does not have a "clinical" component, and CNS involvement may be requested for a variety of activities and committees. It is important that the CNS have leadership support in boundary setting and recognition that not all activities within the CNS's realm need to be performed by the CNS; the oversight of the CNS is adequate for many tasks.

Legislative and regulatory requirements for practice can be an enormous barrier. The National Association of Clinical Nurse Specialists (NACNS) has drafted model statutory and regulatory language in an attempt to assist states to address CNS practice in a consistent fashion.[11] NACNS does not believe that second licensure to practice as a CNS is necessary. The model language (Appendix B) identifies (1) prerequisites to CNS practice, (2) scope of practice for CNSs, and (3) standards and regulations pertaining to CNS practice.[11]

An appropriate CNS/administrator relationship is essential. Successful CNSs are typically highly motivated and self-directed; micromanagement leads to frustration. For maximal effectiveness, the CNS/administrator relationship requires "a unique blend of independence and support along with guidance and creative leadership."[10]

Inability to demonstrate an economic impact through revenue generation or cost savings is another barrier to successful implementation of the CNS role. Rarely do CNSs bill for services,[6] so it is difficult to demonstrate revenue generation, and it is hard to place a dollar amount on the benefit of education, research, consulting, and leadership activities. However, studies have demonstrated that CNSs can affect length of stay, readmission rates, complication rates, medical outcomes, mortality, cost, and patient satisfaction.[12,13] CNSs need to look for nurse- and patient-sensitive outcome measures to demonstrate the value of the role;[14] this area is ripe for future study.

Summary

As an APN with inherent role flexibility, the CNS is in a unique position to improve the quality of nursing and patient care. Although it may be difficult to quantify, implementing the traditional subroles and, potentially, some of the nontraditional subroles of CNS practice can have a dramatic and positive influence on emergency care. In light of the unrelenting change in today's health care environment, a CNS is a valuable member of the ED leadership team.

REFERENCES

1. American Nurses Association. (1996). *Scope and standards of advanced practice registered nursing.* Washington, DC: Author.
2. Lyons, B. L., Davidson, S. B., Beecroft, P. C., Bingle, J., Dayhoff, N., & Ellstrom, K. (1998). *Statement of clinical nurse specialist practice and education.* Glenview, IL: National Association of Clinical Nurse Specialists.
3. Lyons, B. L., & Minarik, P. A. (2001). Statutory and regulatory issues for clinical nurse specialist (CNS) practice. *Clinical Nurse Specialist, 15*(3), 108–114.

4. Redekopp, M. A. (1997). Clinical nurse specialist role confusion: The need for identity. *Clinical Nurse Specialist, 11*(2), 87–91.

5. Moloney-Harmon, P. A. (1999). The synergy model: Contemporary practice of the clinical nurse specialist. *Critical Care Nurse, 19*(2), 101–104.

6. Scott, R. A. (1999). A description of the roles, activities, and skills of clinical nurse specialists in the United States. *Clinical Nurse Specialist, 13*(4), 183–190.

7. Wojner, A. W., & Kite-Powell, D. (1997). Outcomes manager: A role for the advanced practice nurse. *Critical Care Nursing Quarterly, 19*(4), 16–24.

8. Locke, A. M., & Lipkis-Orlando, R. (1993). Organization development: A role for your second-generation clinical nurse specialist. *Nursing Dynamics, 2*(2), 11–12, 14–15.

9. McCaffrey, D. (1991). The unspoken subroles of the clinical nurse specialist. *Clinical Nurse Specialist, 5*(2), 71–72.

10. Boyle, D. M. (1997). Lessons learned from clinical nurse specialist longevity. *Journal of Advanced Nursing, 26*(6), 1168–1174.

11. Lyons, B. L., & Minari, P. A. (2001). National Association of Clinical Nurse Specialists model statutory and regulatory language governing clinical nurse specialist practice. *Clinical Nurse Specialist, 15*(3), 115–120.

12. Maxson, P. M., & Guthmiller, M. L. (1998). A case for the CNS in acute care. *Nursing Management, 29*(9), 35–36.

13. Wheeler, E. C. (1999). The effect of the clinical nurse specialist on patient outcomes. *Critical Care Nursing Clinics of North America, 11*(2), 269–275.

14. Sechrist, K. R., & Berlin, L. E. (1998). Role of the clinical nurse specialist: An integrative review of the literature. *AACN Clinical Issues, 9*(2), 306–324.

Appendix A: Sample CNS Performance Expectations (Job Description)

Clinical Nurse Specialist—Performance Expectations

<u>Job Summary:</u>

The Clinical Nurse Specialist is a Registered Nurse with a Master's degree in a clinical specialty in nursing. The Clinical Nurse Specialist works collaboratively with the health care team to ensure that practice and professional standards are identified and maintained in the delivery of patient care, and that mutually determined patient outcomes are achieved. The job expectations include promoting excellence in patient care, supporting and facilitating professional growth and development, and upholding standards of professionalism.

<u>Standard I:</u>

The Clinical Nurse Specialist functions as an expert clinician/practitioner for a select group of patients.

- Provides direct care to select patients/families as an expert clinician/role model.
- In collaboration with the health care team, facilitates accountability and continuity of care with patients/families.
- Enhances the assessment skills of others as they gather data in a manner that is appropriate to the patient's age, physical ability, intellectual/psychological development, and physical condition.
- Acts as a resource to all members of the health care team related to the provision of patient care, the establishment of appropriate care standards, and the determination of realistic goals for an optimal patient outcome.
- In collaboration with others, assesses the learning needs of specific patient populations and develops patient/family educational tools, classes, or programs.

<u>Standard II:</u>

The Clinical Nurse Specialist enhances the quality of patient care by providing consultation to care providers.

- Consults with the nursing staff and members of the health care team on patient/family care issues.
- Acts as a patient advocate, consulting with the health care team to ensure that mutually determined outcomes are achieved.
- Consults with others on practice issues, ensuring that high standards of professional practice are achieved.
- Participates in clinical improvement efforts.
- Provides consultation on professional issues in nursing and health care, (i.e., Standards of Practice, ethical decision making, documentation) and in clinical specialty area to administrators and others.
- Participates in outreach activities to promote quality care.

<u>Standard III:</u>

The Clinical Nurse Specialist supports and participates in Nursing Research.

- Reads, interprets, and evaluates research for utilization in practice and assists the nursing staff in doing the same.
- Integrates research findings into own practice and the practice of the nursing staff.
- Investigates clinical issues to improve nursing/health care practice, and assists the nursing staff in this process.
- Participates in product evaluation as appropriate.

- Facilitates research conducted by others.
- Facilitates the determination of data needs, data collection, and evaluation of results.

Standard IV:
The Clinical Nurse Specialist facilitates continuing education and orientation of the nursing staff.

- Assesses learning needs of the nursing staff and develops educational strategies to meet those needs.
- Implements, coordinates, or facilitates educational programs that are based on identified learning needs and emerging trends in health care.
- Assures competency of the nursing staff in required skills.
- Facilitates placement and education of nursing students on a specific unit, and may receive adjunct faculty appointment.
- Plans and provides educational programs requested by professional and consumer organizations and assists the nursing staff in doing so.
- In collaboration with others, evaluates educational programs for appropriateness and effectiveness.
- Develops, implements, and evaluates unit-based/specialty orientation.
- Ensures that members of the nursing staff are provided with the skills and resources to develop in their roles.

Standard V:
The Clinical Nurse Specialist demonstrates effective leadership skills when planning, problem solving, and evaluating.

- Develops, implements, and evaluates standards of care, in collaboration with peers, Directors, and the nursing staff.
- Shares accountability for clinical practice in a specialty area, collaborating with peers, Directors, and the nursing staff to ensure standards of care are achieved.
- Provides formal and informal evaluation of the nursing staff, identifying performance issues and facilitating counseling, instruction, or experience as needed.
- In collaboration with peers and the nursing staff, identifies professional practice areas where change is needed and creates and facilitates the change.
- Communicates effectively with all members of the health care team, utilizing negotiation and conflict resolution skills as appropriate.
- In collaboration with the health care team, assists in determining personnel resources to meet patient care requirements.

Standard VI:
The Clinical Nurse Specialist demonstrates accountability for own scholarly and professional activities.

- Participates in appropriate committees and task forces.
- Identifies own learning needs and maintains clinical expertise in area of specialty.
- Engages in activities (i.e., professional organizations, presentations, publications) that contribute to a professional image and positive public relations among nurses, other health care providers, and the public in the region and/or the nation.
- Engages in performance review with CNSs, Directors, Vice Presidents, and nursing staff when appropriate, soliciting feedback regarding performance; determines measurable goals and takes action to achieve those goals.

Appendix B: Model Rules and Regulations for CNS Practice

1. **Title**

   A person who meets all the requirements contained in the definition section may use the title Clinical Nurse Specialist or the initials CNS. No other person is authorized to use the title or initials indicating the person is a CNS.

2. **Definition**

   A Clinical Nurse Specialist (CNS) independently provides theory and research-based care to clients facilitating attainment of health goals, works with nurses to advance nursing practice to improve outcomes cost-effectively, and/or provides clinical expertise to affect system-wide changes in organizations to improve programs of care. The CNS is a registered professional nurse who:

   a. Holds a graduate degree (master's or doctoral) or a post-masters certificate from a program that is recognized by a national nursing accrediting body and that prepares graduates to practice as a CNS.

   b. Holds national certification as a CNS in a designated specialty or in an area pertinent to the designated specialty or met waiver requirements as specified in these rules when there is no certification examination available in the CNS's specialty area.

   c. Meets all other board of nursing requirements to practice as a clinical nurse specialist.

3. **Scope of Practice**

   The CNS provides advanced levels of direct care as defined by the board and assists other nurses and health professionals in both establishing and meeting health goals for individuals and populations of patients. In the provision of direct care services the CNS: 1) integrates advanced knowledge of disease and medical treatments in a holistic assessment of persons while focusing on the diagnosis of symptoms, functional problems, and risk behaviors that have etiologies requiring nursing interventions to prevent, maintain, or alleviate; and 2) utilizes assessment data, research, and theoretical knowledge to design, implement, and evaluate nursing interventions that integrate delegated medical treatments as needed. The CNS is authorized to prescribe or order durable medical equipment when such equipment is a self-care assistive device or assists nurses in the delivery of quality nursing care. Additionally, the CNS who has fulfilled the requirements for prescriptive authority in a specialty area is authorized to prescribe, administer, and distribute medications or pharmaceutical agents in the area of specialty practice. In the provision of indirect patient care services the CNS: 1) serves as a consultant to other nurses and health care professionals in managing highly complex patient care problems or in achieving quality, cost-effective outcomes across settings; 2) serves as a leader in the appropriate use of research in practice innovations that improve patient care; 3) develops, plans, guides, and directs programs of care for populations of patients and provides direction to nursing personnel and others in these programs of care; 4) evaluates patient outcomes and cost-effectiveness of care to identify needs for practice improvements within the clinical specialty or programs; and 5) serves as a leader of multidisciplinary groups in designing and implementing alternative solutions to patient care issues across the continuum of care.

4. **Standards for Clinical Nurse Specialist Scope of Practice**

   a. The CNS, in addition to following the standards for registered nurse practice, is responsible to standards for advanced practice, which include but are not limited to:

      1) Recognizing limits of knowledge and experience and consulting with or referring to other health care providers when appropriate.

2) Providing nursing services that are within the scope of nursing specialty practice for which he or she is educationally prepared and for which competency has been established and maintained through educational preparation such as academic course work, workshops or seminars, other supervised, planned learning that includes theory and clinical experience.

3) Developing jointly derived statements of agreement or jointly derived practice protocols, preprinted orders, or algorithms to facilitate interdependent practice when CNS practice overlaps with the scope of medical practice.

5. **General Regulations Relating to Clinical Nurse Specialists**
   a. Requirements for recognition to practice
      1) Submits evidence to successful completion of master's degree program in a clinical specialty area from an accredited school of nursing. The program's objective must be the preparation of nurses to practice as CNS.
      2) Submits evidence of certification as a CNS in a designated specialty area by a national certifying body approved by the board; OR approval for a waiver of this requirement when no certification exam as a CNS is available in the specialty.
      3) Submits a nonrefundable fee for initial recognition by the board; an incomplete application that remains incomplete shall be considered void after 12 months.

6. **Temporary Recognition to Practice Pending Certification or Approval of Waiver**
   a. Temporary approval to practice pending certification to approval of a waiver may be granted for a period not to exceed 6 months if a graduate of a master's degree program in a clinical specialty area meets the requirements set forth in Section 2(a) and (c);
   b. Evidence shall be submitted that the applicant has applied for and is eligible to take, or has taken, the first available, post-graduation, CNS certification examination given by a national certifying body recognized by the board or has submitted required documents to petition for a waiver; and
   c. Submission of a temporary recognition request application fee approved by the board that is not refundable.

7. **Requirements of Waiver for Initial Recognition**
   Applicant shall submit:
   a. A description of the petitioner's scope of practice to ensure that it is appropriate for CNS role.
   b. A letter from a faculty member who supervised the petitioner during the master's degree program attesting to the petitioner's competence to practice within defined scope of practice; OR a letter from a supervisor verifying petitioner's competence in defined scope of practice; OR a letter from an appropriate collaborating health professional attesting to petitioner's competence in defined scope of practice; and
   c. A form verifying that the petitioner has had a minimum of 500 hours of current practice in specialty area with the previous 2 years (clinical practice time in a master's degree program is applicable); and
   d. An application for a nonrefundable waiver fee as approved by the board.

8. **Requirements for Continuing Recognition to Practice by Certification**
   a. Request for continuing recognition to practice is concurrent with renewal of the registered nurse license.
      1) An applicant shall submit evidence of current certification as a CNS from a certifying body approved by the board; and submit a nonrefundable application fee as specified by the board.

9. **Requirements for Continuing Recognition to Practice by Waiver When There Continues to be No CNS Certification in the Petitioner's Specialty**
   a. Request for continuing recognition to practice is concurrent with renewal of the registered nurse license.
      1) Submits description to petitioner's current scope of practice to ensure that scope is appropriate for CNS role;
      2) Submits a letter from a supervisor or appropriate collaborating professional verifying competence in defined scope of practice; and
      3) Submits a portfolio of exemplar outcomes achieved over time since last waiver—to include data on patient outcomes, nurse outcomes, and/or system outcomes as consistent with the CNS's defined scope of practice and guidelines established by the board.

10. **General Regulations Relating to Prescriptive and Dispensing Authority for Clinical Nurse Specialists**
    a. The CNS who applies for medication prescriptive authority must meet the same requirements as other APNs.

11. **Disciplinary Action on Clinical Nurse Specialists**
    a. The board may deny, suspend, or revoke authority of a CNS to practice based on causes identified (cite statutes/regulations pertinent to registered nurse disciplinary actions) or violation of the standards of CNS practice.
    b. The following actions shall be considered conduct in violation of the standards of nursing practice:
       1) Fraudulently charging the client or any third-party payor;
       2) Using ordering authority without evidence of advanced nursing assessment and establishment of the client/CNS relationship;
       3) Prescribing and/or dispensing medications without specific authority under state law; and
       4) Practicing as a CNS in a specialty area not supported by educational preparation as described in Section 4(a2).
    c. Revocation, suspension, or any other encumbrance of a registered nurse license, or any special authority to practice as a CNS, in another state, territory of the United States, or any foreign jurisdiction may be grounds for denial of authority to practice.

Reprinted with permission from Lyon, B.L., & Minarik, P.A. (2001). National Association of Clinical Nurse Specialists model statutory and regulatory language governing clinical nurse specialist practice. *Clinical Nurse Specialist, 15*(3), 117–118.

8 EMERGENCY NURSE PRACTITIONERS

Vicki A. Keough, RN-CS, PhD, ACNP, CCRN
Frank L. Cole, PhD, RN, CEN, CS, FNP, FAAN, FAANP
Judith A. Jennrich, RN-CS, PhD, ACNP, CCRN
Elda Ramirez, MSN, RN, FNP, CS, CEN

For many, the idea of nurse practitioners (NPs) delivering care in emergency departments (EDs) seems like a new practice model; however, the concept of NPs in emergency care actually originated in the early1970s.[1,2,3] The trajectory for NP practice in EDs has been a tumultuous adventure, with the rise of NP practice in the 1970s, only to see a decline until the 21st century, where NP practice has once again began to flourish. According to the most recent National Sample Survey of Registered Nurses, there are an estimated 102,829 NPs in the United States,[2] most of whom specialize in adult, family, or pediatric health care.[4] One study found that across America, NPs are involved in the care of about 4% of all ED patients.[5] At the same time, it has been estimated that only about 1% of NPs are currently employed in EDs,[1] with only one NP available for every seven NP positions in the United States.[1] Although these statistics may portray a bleak picture of NP practice across the nation, the good news is that NPs working in EDs are growing dramatically and have demonstrated their value in both patient care and cost containment.

It is important to explain early on in this chapter that there are truly no NPs certified as Emergency Nurse Practitioners (ENPs) in the United States at this time because there is no formal certification exam specifically for ENPs. Therefore, most NPs working in EDs currently are either certified as a Family Nurse Practitioner (FNP), an Adult Nurse Practitioner (ANP), a Pediatric Nurse Practitioner (PNP), or an Acute Care Nurse Practitioner (ACNP). Currently there are only two recognized programs in the United States that prepare ENPs through a formal ENP graduate education program; however, there are other programs in the preparation stage. The two current ENP programs are at the University of Texas, Houston,[6] and Loyola University, Chicago.[7]

Although most of the NPs employed in EDs currently possess NP certifications, there is an obvious lack of educational standardization for NPs seeking employment in the unique ED setting. For example, FNP and ANP programs focus on primary care and primary prevention, whereas the ACNP programs tend to focus on caring for the acutely ill adult. PNP programs include both acute and nonacute illnesses, but in the pediatric population only. Obviously, the ENP needs to know how to care for patients of all ages and also needs to be proficient and certified to care for patients with both acute illnesses and chronic diseases. The responsibility is on individual NPs to fill in their educational gaps through mentorship with physicians, experienced NPs already working in EDs, or advanced training and education. The hiring institution expects competent and qualified NPs who are prepared to work in the ED. Some ways the hiring institution can help the NP to further develop ED skills are through skill testing, a solid orientation program, mentorship, and assistance with facilitating practice agreements, credentialing, and privileging. In spite of these issues, research has demonstrated excellent care given by NPs working in EDs across the United States. For the purpose of clarity, the generic term "NPs" will be used throughout this chapter to refer to NPs working in EDs.

In 1991 the Emergency Nurses Association (ENA) issued a position statement supporting advanced practice in emergency nursing[8] (Appendix A). This statement supports and promotes the role of advanced practice in emergency nursing including practice, education, and research. Furthermore, the ENA position statement supports legislative issues promoting third-party reimbursement for advanced nursing practice and for the development and support of graduate emergency nursing programs. The American College of Emergency Physicians supported the practice of nurse practitioners in their publication outlining guidelines for NPs practicing in the emergency department issued in 1995.[9]

Need for ED NPs

With the rising number of ED visits across the nation and a decrease in the number of health care facilities, there is an increased need for more NPs working in EDs. The Centers for Disease Control reported that ED personnel cared for 13 million more patients in 1999 than in 1992,[10] setting a trend for increased ED usage across the nation. The latest national data reveal that ED visits have reported a high of 108 million visits in 2000 with about 70 less hospitals to provide care. Furthermore, this same study reported a 33% increase in waiting times for patients to see a health care provider when presenting with nonurgent conditions.[11] This finding clearly illustrates the need for hospitals to increase their use of NPs to deliver care to ED patients across the United States.

Because 60% to 80% of today's ED patients present with nonurgent or minor medical problems,[10] NPs are qualified to treat the majority of patients with little or no supervision. Considering the length of time patients wait to see a health care professional, the value of the NP becomes increasingly evident.

Nonurgent care is not the only area in which NPs are needed. Hospitals have reported that as many as 47% of ED patients require urgent or emergent care.[11] Several graduate nursing programs prepare NPs to care for the acutely ill patient at the advanced practice level, specifically ACNP and PNP programs. Therefore, depending on the NP's cer-

tification, the NP working in the ED may be fully capable to render care to patients with chronic, episodic, and acute illnesses.

Wilson, Farrell, and Bove[12] conducted a study of NP care at the AtlantiCare Medical Center Program prior to the introduction of NPs to the ED and 3 years after. They found that before NPs were hired, most patients with nonemergent conditions were kept waiting because the physician was treating more seriously ill patients. Patient volumes, acuity, and reimbursement issues prevented the feasibility of adding a second physician. At the time, ED statistics documented prolonged waiting times for patients and large numbers of patients leaving the ED without treatment. After the NPs were introduced to the care mix of the ED, patient wait times decreased, fewer patients left without being seen, there was less patient back-up, and patients reported improved satisfaction.[12] Rhee et al.[13] found similar results in their study conducted in a university medical center, which also reported increased patient satisfaction after the introduction of NPs.

Long waits, untimely care, and a natural tendency for staff to concentrate on acutely ill patients over nonurgent patients are characteristic of most hospital EDs. However, as health care dollars become more competitive, ED managers cannot afford the resultant poor public relations. Consequently, ED administrators are developing innovative, cost-effective services for patients that include the use of NPs.[14]

The benefits of NP staffing in the ED include[15]

- Increased-quality, cost-effective patient care
- Decreased malpractice costs and risks
- Increased ED physician corporate profitability
- Reduced physician contact time with nonurgent patients
- Increased patient satisfaction

NP Efficacy

Dowling and Dudley[15] designed a study to examine NP staffing implications in a busy ED department seeing approximately 45,000 patients per year with a 9% annual census growth rate. The major complaint by patients was the extensive wait time. Findings from the study surprisingly revealed that the majority of nonurgent patients were insured, which made the fast-track area an income-generating area. NPs in the fast-track area could expedite patient flow, thus improving patient satisfaction, increasing visits to the ED, and thereby raising the revenue for the institution. Staffing the fast track with NPs, instead of more expensive emergency physicians, would be cost effective both to the hospital and the physicians and improve community relations with increased patient satisfaction. As a result of this study, the hospital hired an NP for Monday through Friday for the 3 P.M. to 11 P.M. shift. A comprehensive set of written protocols, broad enough to encompass the wide range of patients seen in the ED, was established. A follow-up study is planned to determine the results of this new program.

Another emergency department NP program, established by the AtlantiCare Medical Center,[12] consisted of three part-time and four per diem NPs. The NPs primarily saw all the nonurgent patients. If there were few nonurgent patients, the NPs began the work-up of the urgent patients. Due to the addition of NP positions, the emergency physicians were able to increase their shift times, working 12-hour shifts instead of 10-hour shifts and therefore decrease the number of weekends they were required to work. Patients got quality care more quickly, resulting in a decrease in patient back-up and improved customer satisfaction. NPs also precepted NP students in the ED, acted as resources for the hospital nurses, and supported advanced nursing education. The NPs have also been requested to moonlight in private offices and are held in high esteem within the ED.[12]

In response to complaints of long waits, untimely care, and a tendency to concentrate on acutely ill patients, Vanderbilt University[14] sought a solution to provide more expeditious care without jeopardizing the efficient care of critically ill patients. A fast track, staffed by NPs, was developed to treat patients with low-acuity problems that are easily assessed and quickly treated. Within 6 months of operation, the fast track expanded from 3 days per week to 7 days per week. Staffing consists of two NPs and one receptionist. In its first year of operation, the fast track treated 4,468 patients, an average of 17 patients per day when open. The

number increased to 20 per day after the first 9 months. The number of patients leaving the ED without being seen decreased from an average of 45 per month to an average of 28 per month. Both the ED staff RNs and the emergency physicians are staunch supporters of the ENPs. In a survey of 117 fast-track patients, 96% believed that the care provided by the NP was excellent or very good, and 94% believed that the discharge instructions given by the NP were excellent or very good. Treatment in the fast track was rated at least very good by 87% of the patients; 98% would recommend the service to others. The fast track has increased ED revenue by retaining paying patients and adding follow-up visits.[14]

Other studies have demonstrated that NPs can deliver high-quality care and improve patient satisfaction overall with no difference in patient satisfaction between those treated by emergency physicians and NPs.[16,17] In fact, one study found that NPs scored higher marks than resident physicians in history taking and unplanned return visits requesting discharge advice (or information).[17] Another study conducted at Graduate Hospital in Philadelphia, Pennsylvania, found that although NPs saw a greater number of nonurgent patients than physicians, they also saw a large number of urgent and even emergent patients. Furthermore, the NPs actually saw the same volume of patients over a 1-year period as physicians with very high patient satisfaction results.[18]

Role

The role of NPs in emergency care varies greatly depending on the needs of the institution and the support of the community at large. There are, however, identified responsibilities that are considered basic roles attributed to the NP working in the ED. Cole and Ramirez[19] documented the results of 232 patients seen by NPs in Texas. They found that NPs functioning in EDs and urgent care centers were diagnosing, ordering, and interpreting diagnostic tests and providing independent services, such as wound and orthopedic care. They found most NPs adopt a holistic approach to their patients from the initial assessment and examination through treatment and discharge planning, including education of patients, families, and significant others prior to discharge from the

Table 8-1	
Common Roles of NPs	
■ Provide a model of holistic care	
■ History taking	
■ Perform physical exams	
■ Order diagnostic tests	
■ Diagnose	
■ Generate treatment plans	
■ Prescribe medications	
■ Initiate treatment	
■ Educate patients and families	
■ Provide follow-up care	

emergency department.[20] Table 8-1 lists the common roles of NPs working in the ED.[6,14,16,21]

NPs often become quite proficient in labor-intensive procedures that can alleviate a great deal of time from the hands of the emergency physician. Some examples of the procedures at which NPs are proficient include basic suturing, ordering/interpreting x-rays and laboratory tests, triaging, intubation, laser treatments, application of casts and splints, reduction of dislocations, infiltration of local anesthetics, packing of nose for epistaxis, lumbar punctures, intraosseous insertions, slit lamp examinations, stomach lavage, recording and interpreting of EKGs, digital blocks, simple and complex wound closures, wound debridement, and removal of foreign bodies.[1,19,22,23,24,25]

NPs working in EDs may be employed either by a physician practice group or the hospital, each having its own specific guidelines and responsibilities for the NP.[20] Some NPs work as independent practitioners with a collaborating physician responsible for reviewing charts and implementing sanctioned protocols. Other NPs work in states in which a supervising physician is not mandated by law, and the NP can independently treat minor complaints and injuries without reference to a physician. In many states, NPs are permitted to prescribe medications independently. A comprehensive list of prescriptive authority in each state[25] is available at http://www.medscape.com/viewarticle/440315.

Another role of the NP is to work in collaboration with an ED physician caring for the critically ill patient. ENPs must be prepared to deliver care to all levels and types of emergency patients. They must have the diagnostic and therapeutic skills to administer lifesaving interventions.[6] In treating the acutely ill patient, the NP works within a collaborative framework with the medical staff.

Education

Education of the NP in emergency care needs to be broad based, encompassing care of patients of all ages and diseases, including victims of violence and nonintentional injuries.[1] The NP working in emergency care has to be able to prioritize patient problems without the benefit of long-term history, treat the most immediate problem, and determine whether the injury is self-limiting or requires referral to continuing care.[1] A strong clinical ED background along with a rigorous graduate education can prepare the NP to function in the ED and provide safe, comprehensive, and competent care. As stated at the chapter onset, most NPs working in EDs have graduated from an FNP, PNP, ANP, or ACNP program. A disadvantage of these programs is that they do not focus specifically on emergency care, and therefore graduates from these programs need to find other avenues to obtain the clinical and theoretical expertise they require to practice in a busy ED. Two established ENP programs aim to prepare the ENP to step into an ED role immediately after graduation.[6,7] Regardless of what type of basic graduate education the NP receives, continuing education is a must for all NPs.[7,13] Continuing education can be obtained through national Emergency Nurses Association, American Association of Critical-Care Nurses or NP conferences, online, through journal readings, or by attendance at local continuing educational offerings.

The current goals of the University of Texas and Loyola University, Chicago, ENP programs include (1) preparing APNs to function efficiently and effectively in all levels and types of EDs, (2) developing the diagnostic and therapeutic skills to intervene in life-threatening conditions, and (3) providing care to clients of all ages.[6,7]

These two ENP masters' degree programs require approximately 48 to 49 semester hours of post-BSN study and more than 600 hours of clinical practice prior to graduation. Although ANP, FNP, PNP, and ACNP programs also require similar theoretical and practical requirements prior to graduation, the content of those programs do not specifically focus on ED care.

Another educational model recently introduced for NPs wishing to advance their experience and education as an ENP is a post-MSN program. This model was introduced in 2000 at the University of San Diego, California.

Certification

Certification attests that one has obtained a defined body of knowledge in a respective area. In most states, a nurse practitioner must be certified in his or her area of specialty by a national certification entity to practice as an NP. If a certification existed for ENPs and one became certified, this would indicate to the public that the certified ENP possessed the knowledge necessary for practice in the ED. Because there is no specialty certification for ENPs, graduate students must be prepared for a more general exam. Currently NPs working in the ED have graduated from an accredited NP program and passed their respective certification exam. Ideally, one day there will be a national certification examination that specifically addresses the knowledge and practice expertise of ENPs.

Future of ENPs

As Barbara Safriet stated, "The boundaries of responsibility for nurses are not shifting more rapidly simply because of increased demands for health services. The functions of nurses are changing primarily because nurses have demonstrated their competence to perform a greater variety of functions."[26] NPs have risen to the occasion and have demonstrated their proficiency and expertise in the delivery of care to ED patients. Not only have NPs demonstrated their ability to deliver competent care, but they have also demonstrated cost savings to institutions, improvement in patient satisfaction, and overall improvement in ED care. The future for NPs in the ED looks bright. In the future, EDs will boast about their efficient use of NPs and physicians, both professionals combining their education and skills to provide the best care possible to the community they serve. There will come a time, hope-fully sooner rather than later, when NPs will be a part of every "best-practice model" for EDs across the country.

REFERENCES

1. Curry, J. L. (1994). Nurse practitioners in the emergency department: Current issues. *Journal of Emergency Nursing, 20*(3), 207–212.
2. Spratley, E., Johnson, A., Sochalski, J., Fritz, M., & Spencer, W. (2000). *The registered nurse population: Findings from the national sample survey of registered nurses.* Washington, DC: U.S. Department of Health and Human Services, Health Resources and Service Administration Bureau of Health Professions, Division of Nursing 2000. Retrieved November 26, 2002 from http://www.bhpr.hrsa.gov/healthworkforce/rnsurvey/rnss1.htm
3. Fincke, M. K. (1975). A new dimension in emergency nursing. *Journal of Emergency Nursing, 1*(5), 45–52.
4. American Nurses Association. (1992). *Executive summary. A meta-analysis of process of care, clinical outcomes and cost effectiveness of nurses in primary care roles: Nurse practitioners and nurse midwives.* Washington, DC: Author.
5. Hooker, R. S., & McCaig, L. (1975). Emergency department use of physician assistants and nurse practitioners: A national survey. *American Journal of Emergency Medicine, 14*(3), 245–254.
6. Cole, F. L., & Ramirez, E. (1996). The emergency nurse practitioner: An educational model. *Journal of Emergency Nursing, 23*(2), 112–115.
7. Keough, V. (2001). Emergency nurse practitioners lighten patient loads, boost satisfaction. *Nursing Spectrum, 14,* 4.
8. Emergency Nurses Association. (2000). *Advanced practice in emergency nursing (position statement).* Retrieved November 27, 2002 from http://www.ena.org/about/position/advancedpractice.asp
9. American College of Emergency Physicians. (2000). *Guidelines on the role of nurse practitioners in emergency departments.* Retrieved November 26, 2002 from http://www.acep.org/1,583,0.html
10. National Center for Health Statistics. (2002). *Trends in hospital emergency department utilization: United States, 1992–1999.* Hyattsville, MD: U.S. Department of Health and Human Services, Centers for Disease Control and Prevention. Retrieved December 4, 2002 from http://www.cdc.gov/nchs/products/pubs/pubd/series/sr13/150-141/sr13_150.htm
11. National Center for Health Statistics. (2002). *Visits to the emergency department increase nationwide. National hospital ambulatory medical care survey: 2000 emergency department summary.* Hyattsville, MD: U.S. Department of Health and Human Services, Centers for Disease Control and Prevention. Retrieved December 4, 2002 from http://www.cdc.gov/nchs/releases/02news/emergency.htm

12. Wilson, C., Farrell, M., & Bove, S. (1994). Emergency department nurse practitioners: The AtlantiCare medical center program in review. *Journal of Emergency Nursing, 20*(3), 195–198.

13. Rhee, K. J., & Dermyer, A. L. (1995). Patient satisfaction with a nurse practitioner in a university emergency service. *Annals of Emergency Medicine, 26*(2), 130–131.

14. Covington, C., Erwin, T., & Sellers, F. (1992). Implementation of a nurse practitioner-staffed fast track. *Journal of Emergency Nursing, 18*(2), 124–131.

15. Dowling, D., & Dudley, W. (1995). Nurse practitioners: Meeting the ED's needs. *Nursing Management, 26*(1), 48C–48E, 48J.

16. Chang, E., Daly, J., Hawkins, A., McGirr, J., Fielding, K., Hemmings, L., et al. (1999). An evaluation of the nurse practitioner role in a major rural emergency department. *Journal of Advanced Nursing, 30*(1), 260–268.

17. Sakr, M., Angus, J., Perrin, J., Nixon, C., Nicholl, J., & Wardrope, J. (1999). Care of minor injuries by emergency nurse practitioners or junior doctors: A randomised controlled trial. *Lancet, 354,* 1321–1326.

18. Blunt, E. (1998). Role and productivity of nurse practitioners in one urban emergency department. *Journal of Emergency Nursing, 24*(3), 234–239.

19. Cole, F., & Ramirez, E. (1999). Evaluating an emergency nurse practitioner educational program for its relevance to the role. *Journal of Emergency Nursing, 25*(6), 547–550.

20. Cole, F. L., Ramirez, E., & Mickanin, J. (1999). ED nurse practitioners' employment by a physician group versus hospital: Pros and cons. *Journal of Emergency Nursing, 25*(3), 183–186.

21. Woolwich, C. (1992). A wider frame of reference. *Nursing Times, 88*(46), 34–36.

22. Marshall, J. (1997). Protocols and emergency nurse practitioners. *Nursing Times, 93*(14), 58–60.

23. Dimond, B. (1995). The scope of professional practice and the accident and emergency nurse. *Accident and Emergency Nursing, 23*(2), 105–107.

24. Cole, F. L., & Ramirez, E. (2000). Activities and procedures performed by nurse practitioners in emergency care settings. *Journal of Emergency Nursing, 26*(5), 455–463.

25. Byrne, W. (2002). *U.S. nurse practitioner prescribing laws: A state-by-state survey.* Retrieved November 26, 2002 from http://www.medscape.com/viewarticle/440315

26. Safriet, B. (1992). Health care dollars and regulatory sense: The role of advanced practice nursing. *Yale Journal on Regulation, 9,* 417–418.

Appendix A
EMERGENCY NURSES ASSOCIATION POSITION STATEMENTS

ADVANCED PRACTICE IN EMERGENCY NURSING

Introduction

Clinical Nurse Specialists (CNS) and Nurse Practitioners (NP) have been established as Advanced Practice Nurses since 1965 (ANA, 1995). The Emergency Nurses Association defines an advanced practice nurse (APN) as one who minimally: (1) has completed a Master's degree in a specialty area of nursing; and (2) is clinically active in the specialty area. Not only are these nurses seen as clinical patient care experts, but expanded roles of advanced practice nurses involve leadership/administration, consultation, education, and research (ENA, 1996).

Currently, the role of the emergency nurse in advanced practice is under utilized due to many factors. These factors include:

- Lack of awareness of their functions, qualifications and abilities
- Limited number of graduate emergency nursing programs
- Lack of research related to the cost saving outcomes that APNs produce
- Varied use of advanced practice titles
- Differences in state nurse practice acts
- Different levels of administrative support for the advanced practice nurse in emergency care
- Economic/financial crisis in health care and health care institutions
- Limitation and practice in relation to varying state boards of nursing regulations

Association Position

ENA supports and promotes the use of advanced practice nurses in emergency care.

ENA believes specialty organizations have the right and responsibility to define advanced nursing practice and to institute appropriate certifying procedures.

ENA supports efforts that make advanced nursing practice more uniform and more clearly defined.

ENA recognizes the "Scope of Practice for the Nurse Practitioner in the Emergency Care Setting" (ENA, 1999) for the definition of the responsibilities, functions, roles, and skills of Nurse Practitioners in emergency care.

ENA recognizes and supports the State Boards of Nurse Examiners as the governing body, and each State Nurse Practice Act as the authority to delineate reporting and licensing regulations.

ENA supports all legislative efforts to promote third party reimbursement, prescriptive authority, and autonomy for advanced nursing practice.

ENA supports the establishment of standards and clear criteria for credentialing of the advanced practice nurse in the emergency care setting.

ENA supports federal, state, local, and private grants and appropriations for the development and support of graduate emergency nursing programs.

Rationale

Emergency health care systems have been adversely affected by the current crisis in health care. This has created a need for innovative and cost effective approaches to the care of emergency patients. An advanced practice emergency nurse is uniquely prepared to develop and apply theory, research, and standards of care that enhance patient outcomes.

References

American Nurses Association (ANA). (1995). *Nursing's social policy statement.* Washington, DC: Author.

Cole, F.L., Ramirez, E., & Luna-Gonzales, H. (1999). *Scope of practice for the nurse practitioner in the emergency care setting.* Des Plaines, IL: ENA.

Emergency Nurses Association (ENA). (1996). *Advanced nursing practice manual.* Des Plaines, IL: Author.

Bibliography

Mundinger, M., Kane, R., & Lenz, E. (2000). Primary care outcomes in patients treated by nurse practitioners or physicians: a randomized trial. *Journal of American Medical Association, 283*(1), 59–68.

O'Neil, E. (1995, November). Critical Challenges: Revitalizing the health professions for the twenty-first century. *The third report of The Pew Health Professions Commission.*

U.S. Office of Technology Assessment. (1986). *Health technology case study 37: Nurse practitioners, physician assistants, and certified nurse midwives: A policy analysis.* U.S. Government Printing Office.

Developed: 1991.

Revised and approved by the ENA Board of Directors: September, 1993.

Revised and approved by the ENA Board of Directors: August, 1994.

Revised and approved by the ENA Board of Directors: September, 1996.

Revised and approved by the ENA Board of Directors: July, 1998.

Revised and approved by the ENA Board of Directors: September, 2000.

9   Practice Protocols/Guidelines

Lynn Scarbrough, RN, MSN, ACNP

Emergency department (ED) advanced practice nurses (APNs) provide direct patient care over a wide range of competencies on a vast continuum of severity of injury and illness. It is essential to provide research-based, quality care. Practice protocols or guidelines enable APNs, whether nurse practitioners (NPs) or clinical nurse specialists (CNSs) to implement their role within a defined, standardized framework. These protocols/guidelines are research or evidence based, allowing practice within widely held standards of care.

Appropriate protocols or guidelines for APNs are required by many states. *The Nurse Practitioner: The American Journal of Primary Healthcare* publishes annual updates of each state's legislative regulations on advanced nursing practice. Practice protocols differ from guidelines in many ways. It is important for APNs to understand these differences in an effort to design and implement what is most appropriate or required for each practice setting. In some settings, the APN will want to follow guidelines, whereas in other settings, protocols will be required.

Practice Protocols

A practice protocol is a step-by-step process written for a specific clinical situation to govern aspects of care requiring medical authorization and to allow for standardization of care. The protocol should specifically state circumstances in which physician collaboration is required. Protocols are arbitrary and followed without deviation. Well-written protocols are clinically relevant, research or evidence based, and logically sequenced. Protocols should be developed by a multidisciplinary team and be clear, without ambiguity.[1] The protocols should apply to most patient care situations and meet the needs of a general target patient population.[2]

Practice protocols may be presented in flowcharts, diagrams, or algorithmic formats. Alternatively, protocols can be drafted in the well-known SOAP (subjective, objective, assessment, and plan) format. They should be frequently reevaluated and updated to maintain clinical relevance as new scientific data emerges. Several prepublished books containing protocols exist, such as *Nurse Practitioner Protocols, Ambulatory Care Procedures for the Nurse Practitioner,* and *Directory of Clinical Practice Guidelines: Titles, Sources and Updates.* The American College of Emergency Physicians publishes an extensive manual of protocols specific to ED practice.[3] An example of a practice protocol is shown in Appendix A.

Guidelines

Guidelines are a broader, more flexible approach to converting evidence-based knowledge into clinical care that allow the APN to customize care based on unique clinical situations.[2] Guidelines, like protocols, include circumstances requiring physician consultation. Most often, statements such as "relative indications," "generally appropriate or inappropriate practices," or "drugs/procedures of choice" constitute a guideline. Protocols specify instructions that must be followed exactly, whereas guidelines provide general recommendations. For an example of an ED practice guideline, see Appendix B.

Components of Practice Protocols

Practice protocols consist of several components (see Table 9-1). First, the problem must be de-

Table 9-1
Practice Protocol Components[1]
<ul><li>Background information or definition of the problem</li><li>Subjective data (questions to ask)</li><li>Objective data (physical exam, diagnostics, procedures)</li><li>Assessment (diagnosis, differential diagnoses)</li><li>Plan (treatment, medications, referrals, consultation)</li><li>Patient/family education</li><li>Follow-up</li><li>References</li></ul>

fined or clearly stated. This can be achieved by defining the problem as a physiologic state or chief complaint. For example, a set of inclusion criteria that defines asthma can be established. When a patient presents meeting the inclusion criteria for asthma, the protocol is utilized.

Next, the protocol outlines what subjective data must be obtained from the patient or other sources. Depending on the type of situation being addressed in the protocol, risk factors may also be included. The extent of this portion of the protocol depends on the severity and complexity of the pathophysiology involved. In other words, a urinary tract infection protocol would consume less time and be more streamlined in this section than would an acute myocardial infarction protocol.

Objective data includes the minimum and usual physical exam, diagnostic tests, and procedures required for safe care. Tests such as sophisticated radiographic scans that may not be available at off hours or laboratory diagnostics that are not available in all site settings are not included.

The assessment and differential diagnoses process assists the APN in considering other possible diagnoses as well as ensuring thorough documentation and evaluation of the patient. Once the assessment and diagnosis phase is completed, the APN uses the protocols to help form the comprehensive plan of care.

The plan outlines treatments that are indicated by research data, best practices, or evidence-based practice. Prescribing guidelines are included as well as directions for referral and consultation. Although requirements for direct consultation with

physicians must be very clearly delineated, prescribing patterns, treatments, follow-up instructions, and patient education are addressed flexibly enough to allow for APN discretion. Education requirements for the patient and/or the patient's family are delineated, such as providing asthma educational brochures as part of an asthma protocol. Follow-up care instruction should also remain a flexible part of the protocol. Specific time frames should be recommended, with exact follow-up directed by the APN.

References must be current and regularly updated. Ideally, a multidisciplinary team drafts the protocols, and each team member gives input concerning their area of expertise. This allows protocols to be used by more than one discipline. For example, a respiratory therapist should be consulted while drafting an asthma protocol, not only to provide expertise but also to promote cooperation and facilitate team-oriented patient care.

Keeping abreast of changes in clinical practice is essential. Updating protocols based on current scientific research or changes in the epidemiology of a region is also very important. Protocols are evaluated and signed by those involved, usually the ED physician or physician group, at least annually. The date of review must be clearly documented.

Pros and Cons of Practice Protocols

Practice protocols provide clear, concise treatment plans that can be reassuring to those new to the novice APN and to other health care providers who are unfamiliar with an APN's capabilities. Protocols tend to control cost and are especially helpful in streamlining care. It is not uncommon for new APN programs to start with protocol-driven practices, only to convert to guidelines when the "waters have been proven" and the APN role has been established as safe and cost effective with high levels of patient satisfaction. In states in which protocols are required, this is not an option.

Practice protocols are frequently used by the legal system as a standard for measuring a clinician's practice.[4] Practice protocols are usually developed with the classic patient presentation in mind. Because all patients do not present this way, it may be appropriate to deviate from a protocol. When poor outcomes occur in these situations, the practitioner may be accused of deviating from the standard, thus implying liability. Therefore, it is recommended that the APN consult with a physician when deviation from protocols occur and carefully document the reasons for the change.

Legal Aspects of Practice Protocols/Guidelines

Strategies for reducing liability when practice protocols are required include developing minimalist protocols, updating protocols as knowledge develops, accounting for practice variables, and requiring minimum safety standards.[4] Minimalist protocols tend to be very simple and apply to a certain problem or set of symptoms in all circumstances. Protocols should ensure the minimums of safe care, not the maximum for ideal care. Raising a standard of care is a set-up for legal consequences.

Once the protocols are drafted, they must be followed without deviation. If the protocol is breached, clear documentation of the reasons for the deviation should be included in the patient record.[4] If a protocol is no longer in use, a "retired" date should be documented. The protocol should be archived for the states' mandated statute of limitations in case a lawsuit occurs. In this event, the APN has some evidence that the care provided was within the scope of the protocol at that time.[1]

Summary

Practice guidelines and protocols can facilitate safe, streamlined, and high-quality patient care. If written in a language that allows for flexibility and case-by-case judgment, protocols and guidelines can be very useful if not otherwise mandated by state law. Most states do require a minimum set of practice guidelines delineating a standard of care in a given situation. Whenever possible, broader and more flexible guidelines should prevail to allow the APN to utilize the unique qualifying attributes of this highly skilled role.

REFERENCES

1. Paul, S. (1999). Developing practice protocols for advanced practice nursing. *AACN Clinical Issues, 10*(3), 343–355.
2. Gawlinski, A. (1995). Practice protocols: Development and use. *Critical Care Nursing Clinics of North America, 7*(1), 17–23.
3. American College of Emergency Physicians. (2002). *Practice resources.* Retrieved October 10, 2002 from http://www.acep.org
4. Moniz, D. M. (1992). The legal danger of written protocols and standards of practice. *Nurse Practitioner, 17*(9), 58–60.

Appendix A
Example of a Practice Protocol

Strep Pharyngitis

"S" Chief complaint may include:
1. Throat pain, increased with swallowing, pain below jaw line
2. Fever (low grade to 102°F+)
3. Swollen, tender neck nodes
4. Sudden onset
5. Recent exposure
6. Headache
7. Fatigue
8. Decreased appetite

"O" Findings may include:
1. Tympanic membranes may be injected
2. Throat erythematous, tonsils swollen with whitish exudate. Tonsils may be beefy red without exudate.
3. Bilateral anterior cervical lymphadenopathy
4. Temperature 100°F+

"A" Strep Pharyngitis:
Differential Diagnosis: Viral Pharyngitis
Infectious Mononucleosis
Peritonsillar Abscess

"P" Plan may include:
1. Strep screen or throat culture. If positive or high level of suspicion, treat with:

   A. Penicillin VK 250 mg QID × 10 days, if not PCN allergic
   B. Amoxicillin 250 mg q 8 hrs × 10 days
   C. Erythromycin 250 mg QID × 10 days if PCN allergic or PCE 333 TID × 10 days
   D. Zithromax per weight
   E. Consult physician for injectable antibiotic

2. Consult physician for severe swelling of tonsils or difficulty swallowing (R/O peritonsillar abscess)

Patient Education:
1. Rest, push oral fluids. Tylenol® for fever and pain; warm saltwater gargles TID.
2. Notify patient to call physician if persistent fever and pain after 24 hours despite Tylenol®, difficulty swallowing, or other concerns.
3. Notify patient he/she no longer contagious 24 hours after initiating antibiotic therapy
4. If culture positive, will need full 10 days of treatment
5. Refer symptomatic family members for culture

Revised 3/1/98

Reprinted with permission from N. Ryan, MD and R. Thomas, MD, Emergency Care Group, Lake Zurich, IL.

Appendix B
Example of a Practice Guideline

NP Evaluation and Management of Emergency Department/Treatment Center Patients

Medical screening exams may be performed on many patients presenting to the treatment centers, emergency department and annex by the nurse practitioner on duty. Patients evaluated and treated by the nurse practitioner will be discussed with the Emergency Department Attending Physician, who will cosign the medical record prior to the patient's discharge. The Emergency/Attending Physician must examine selected patients, delineated below.

The Supervising Attending Emergency Physician on duty must be consulted by the Nurse Practitioner and the Supervising Attending Emergency Physician must examine the patient under the following clinical circumstances:

- Prior to the performance of invasive procedures such as incision and drainage of paronychia, abscesses, evacuation of subungual hematomas, soft tissue foreign body removal, and joint reduction and the ordering of the following medication for emergency department, annex or treatment center patients:

    Narcotic analgesics
    Sedative hypnotics
    Major tranquilizers

- Prior to the repair of lacerations of the hand and face and any laceration associated with visible contamination, a foreign body and/or nerve, vascular or tendonous injury
- For the review of x-rays and laboratory data (with the exception of urinalyses and streptococcal screens of the throat) prior to the discharge of the patient
- Prior to the discharge of patients with animal and human bites, head injury, abdominal pain, fractures, and ocular complaints
- Prior to the discharge of patients returning within 72 hours with the same or similar chief complaint
- Prior to the discharge of children aged 36 months or younger with a fever of 102°F or more with or without a source
- Prior to discharge of children under 6 months of age with fever, abdominal pain, and irritability

The Supervising Attending Emergency Physician on duty with the nurse practitioner will initiate the management of patients presenting to the emergency department, annex, and treatment centers with respiratory distress, head injury with GCS < 15, multiple system trauma, and high-risk chest pain.

Revised 3/02

Reprinted with permission from N. Ryan, MD, and R. Thomas, MD, Emergency Care Group, Lake Zurich, IL.

10

EPISODIC CARE

T. Smith, RN, MS, CS, FNP-C

The roles for the advanced practice nurse (APN) have expanded over the last 10 to 15 years to include the emergency department (ED) and other areas outside the ED, which have evolved in response to market needs and desires. The Emergency Nurses Association inclusively named these outside care arenas Episodic Care Centers (ECCs) in its 1999 resolution.[1] Table 10-1 lists titles used to designate ECCs. Many ECCs have evolved in response to diminished patient satisfaction with long ED wait times. The patient of the early 21st century demands rapid treatment, the patient may not have an established primary care provider, or primary care provider availability may not be conducive to the patient's life schedule. In some areas, ECCs provide care to families new to an area or in heavily vacationed areas.[2] Episodic care centers can help relieve overcrowding in the ED by allowing nonurgent patients to be seen rapidly. They are frequently adjacent to the ED, but many are freestanding centers and can be located in urban, suburban, rural, or frontier areas.[3]

The role of the ECC in the larger scope of the health care system is still evolving, placing APNs in a prime position to establish this as one of their future roles. APNs, especially those with an ED background, are perfectly suited to staff ECCs in either a solo or a collaborative role with other health care providers. The role of the APN in the ECC spans all domains of practice, including clinical, education, administrative, research, and professional. As with all APN roles, the percentage of time devoted to each domain will vary with the position and practice site.

The clinical role for an APN in the ECC will usually take the major percentage of time commitment. The role is very dependent on the practice environment and collaborative role of physicians and nursing staff. If the APN is the sole provider at the site, it will require a strong clinical background. Ideally a background in emergency care or a similar environment will aid the APN in identifying difficult diagnoses and knowing when and how to appropriately transfer a patient to a higher level of care. Having protocols can help the APN with these difficult decisions. Table 10-2 provides a list of diagnoses frequently encountered in an ECC. Some remote ECC sites have a physician available for consultation by telephone or telemedicine. Sites also vary in clinical resources such as laboratory and radiology availability. The spectrum of availability spans from no diagnostic resources to full resources on-site. When resources

Table 10-1	
Titles Used to Designate ECCs	
Fast Track	Immediate Care Clinic
Ambulatory Care Center	Ambulatory Medical Clinic
Nonurgent Care Center	Urgent Clinic
Ambulatory Urgent Care Center	Urgent Care Center or Clinic
Convenient Care Center	Primary Care Clinic
Episodic Care Center	Freestanding Emergency Clinic
Ambulatory Primary Care Center	Ambulatory Immediate Care Clinic

(Note: *Center* and *clinic* are frequently used interchangeably.)

Table 10-2

	Frequent Diagnoses in ECCs	
Corneal abrasion	Earache	Toothache or mouth blisters
Conjunctivitis	Sore throat	Fever
Mild upper respiratory infection	Acute or chronic sinusitis	Cough without COPD (chronic obstructive pulmonary disease)
Hay fever	Asthma	Request for tetanus shot
Minor skin infections, sores, rash, or sunburn	Minor contusions, lacerations, abrasions, or avulsions	Suture removal or wound check
Puncture wound	Lice or scabies infestation	Insect bites or stings
Nausea, vomiting, diarrhea	Mild dehydration	Constipation of < 3 days
Minor fractures	Joint pain or low back pain without neurological deficit	Foot problems (blisters, pain, ingrown toenails, subungual hematomas)
Muscle aches	Chronic recurrent hematuria	Acute urinary tract infection
Minor rectal pain, itching, or bleeding	Minor vaginal bleeding or discharge	Sexually transmitted disease exposure
Headaches without deficit	Anxiety	Pregnancy testing

Note: This list is not meant to be exclusive.

are not available, the APN must rely on referring patients for follow-up care. For example, if radiology is off-site, patients may be required to drive to another site and return to the ECC with the x-rays for the APN to interpret. Or the APN may rely on further referral to another physician at another site. This requires the APN to be explicit in patient instructions and to ensure patient understanding. Written patient instruction should always be utilized. Having off-site diagnostic resources may increase concerns of the APN regarding liability. Patient follow-up from the ED has always been a concern to providers, and this concern is the same in ECCs. See Table 10-3 for questions to ask yourself before working in an ECC.

Many of the concerns in an off-site solo practice environment are resolved when the APN works in an ECC adjacent to an ED. Because the diagnostic resources are available in the ED-based ECC, this may result in an increase in patient acuity. Physicians practicing in an adjacent ED may be too busy at times to offer consultation on patient issues, which leaves the APN to function alone. The APN must keep this in mind when interviewing for a position or when writing a role description or collaborative practice agreement.

Another large portion of the APN domain in the ECC encompasses the educator role for patients and staff. Patient education will often include not only discharge instruction but also "teaching moments" (M. Silliker, personal communication, April, 2002). Much of the APN domain for patient education incorporates preventative care, and every patient encounter is an opportunity for teaching. For example, the diabetic patient who comes to the ECC for a sinus infection may not have had an annual vision exam or physical, making the ECC encounter a "teaching moment" to remind the patient of this need.

Staff education in the ECC may be delegated to the APN as part of the role, usually because of the advanced education level in nursing. This can be a challenge because ECCs are staffed with a variety of workers, including registered nurses (RNs), licensed practical nurses, care technicians, emergency medical technicians—basic and advanced, medical assistants, and those trained on the job. According to the MacLean ECC benchmark data, RNs employed in ECCs vary between 0 (14%) and 33 (1%).[2] Because most centers are open between 12 and 16 hours per day 7 days per week, many are staffed with care providers other than RNs. This creates a challenging issue for the APN

Table 10-3	
Questions to Ask Yourself Prior to Working in an ECC	

Do you function well independently?

Do you have strong clinical skills as an APN?

Are you confident in your decisions?

How and when will you access a collaborating physician?

Do you know the referral physicians you will be using in the area?

What diagnostic testing is available to help with clinical diagnosis? Are you comfortable and confident in your ability to interpret tests (e.g., laboratory or radiology tests)?

What follow-up system is in place to ensure that patients continue their care beyond the ECC?

Have you successfully completed advanced cardiac life support, trauma nursing core course, emergency nursing pediatric course, or pediatric advanced life support?

What, if any, emergency equipment and supplies are available at the ECC? Are there protocols in place to use in an emergency, and does everyone know about them?

Are you able to delegate tasks easily and explicitly?

Do you know the scope of practice and rules and regulations regarding RN and APN practice in your state?

Do you have a strong professional and collaborative group you can rely on for support and to use as a sounding board for difficult APN practice questions?

and can require assessment of knowledge levels dependent on the topic being discussed. Many APNs provide both formal and informal education for ECC staffs. There are many resources available to assist the APN in providing formal education and in understanding the role of educator (see Chapter 11). Informal education for nursing staff frequently will be related to cases encountered in the ECC and may lead to discussions and further formal education classes. The staff education level will affect the APN in other ways directly related to patient care. If staff does not have skills to assist in patient care, the APN may have to provide this care, which directly affects the number of patients for which the APN is able to provide care. For example, if the APN needs to start and monitor IV fluids, draw labs, run labs, and give injections and medications, this will directly affect the APN's productivity level. This may open many opportunities for the APN to teach staff to perform some of these functions. Some education functions are obvious, and many more will be identified over time. Staff acceptance, openness, and willingness to learn greatly affect this part of the APN's role.

The APN should also be keenly aware of the state scope of practice laws and delegation rules. Most states do not allow RNs or APNs to delegate care

that involves assessment. Any care that requires the RN or APN to perform the basics of an exam (inspection, auscultation, percussion, or palpation) and interpret those findings cannot be delegated. Many ECC staff may not understand this or have always been allowed to perform beyond their scope, which can lead the APN to another staff education need.

The administrative role of the APN is often openly identified in the job description or during the interview. Many APN positions in an ECC have an administrator function. An early administrative task to perform is writing one's collaborative practice agreement. Other tasks may include budgetary tasks, ordering supplies, writing policy and procedures, writing grants, staff evaluations, and ensuring OSHA and Clinical Laboratory Improvement Act compliance. Just performing the administrative tasks associated with a medication sample closet can be very time consuming and labor intensive. If there is an administrative component to the position, the APN should have office management time delegated during the daily schedule or weekly at a minimum.

The domain of research for the ECC APN may involve bringing research into practice or interpreting research for patients and staff. The APN should be studious in reviewing current research to interpret the findings for patients and staff. In the 21st century most media sources will report current medical research, which places the APN in the forefront as an expert to answer questions and explain how the findings relate to patients and their care. Current research will affect clinical practice daily in prescribing medications and ordering diagnostic tests and therapies. Keeping current in pharmaceutical research and new medications is a daunting task, and the APN may find it professionally enhancing to sign up for medication listservs, subscribe to medication newsletters, and attend professional continuing education events frequently.

Attending continuing education events is often enhanced by membership in professional organizations. Being a member of one's professional organization can be especially rewarding for APNs in the ECC environment because it can offer opportunities to discuss practice issues, protocols, and research. Because many APNs are alone in a practice, joining a professional organization provides the opportunity to keep current with professional issues and changes.

In summary, the roles of the APN in the ECC environment can provide a fulfilling career by including multiple aspects of the APN role with a major focus on the clinical practice. A background in emergency nursing enhances the independence an ECC offers to an APN.

REFERENCES

1. Emergency Nurses Association. (1999). *Episodic care centers (ECC), e.g., urgent care centers/fast track, etc.* (Resolution number 99-02). Des Plaines, IL: Author.
2. MacLean, S. (2002). ENA releases new study on episodic care centers. *ENA Connection, 26,* 12–13.
3. North American Association for Ambulatory Urgent Care (NAFAC). (2002). *Definition of urgent care medicine and scope of service.* Retrieved April 2, 2002 from http://www.nafac.com.

PART FOUR EDUCATOR

11

TEACHING STRATEGIES

Rebecca A. Steinmann, RN, MS, CEN, CCRN, CCNS

Education of patients and families, the community, nurses, and other health care professionals is an integral component of the advanced practice nursing (APN) role. Through informal means (e.g., bedside teaching; role modeling; and dialoguing with patients, families, and staff) and in more structured formats (e.g., in-services, lectures, and workshops), APNs facilitate learning by sharing their knowledge and advanced clinical skills with others. The steps of designing an effective teaching strategy parallel those of the nursing process: (1) assessing the problem, (2) diagnosing/analyzing the data, (3) planning and implementing an intervention, and (4) evaluating the response. An understanding of needs assessment, adult learning principles, and instructional design will enable the APN to promote expertise in clinical practice and enhance patient outcomes through effective educational programming.

Assessing the Need for an Educational Intervention

The APN is commonly consulted to assess and identify the learning needs of patients, families, and staff; conduct formal and informal education programs for patients, staff, and the community on various topics; ensure compliance with regulatory mandates (e.g., Joint Commission on Accreditation of Healthcare Organizations requirements for annual review of fire safety and infection control); and address individual performance problems. The starting point for developing meaningful teaching strategies is a clear understanding of the target group's specific need(s).

A need may be defined as a discrepancy or a gap between actual performance (i.e., what is) and de-

sired or optimal performance (i.e., what should be). Burton and Merrill[1] identified six categories of needs to be considered when conducting an educational needs assessment:

1. Normative needs: An individual or group fails to meet established national standards.
2. Comparative needs: Individuals or groups with similar characteristics do not perform to the same external measure.
3. Felt needs: An individual has a desire or want to improve either his or her performance or that of the target audience.
4. Expressed needs: A felt need is turned into action.
5. Anticipated or future needs: Assessing demands of the future.
6. Critical incident need: Failures that rarely occur, but have significant consequences when they happen.

Numerous strategies can be used to assess learning needs. Actual performance can be directly observed while making rounds or by staffing in the department. Skill inventories and checklists, pretests, and documentation audits may identify unmet normative or comparative needs. Written questionnaires and surveys, interviews, informal discussions, and focus groups are frequently used to assess felt needs and identify educational interests. A sample formal learning needs assessment tool is shown in Figure 11-1. Patient letters and comments, program evaluation comments, leadership and unit meetings, committee reports, quality improvement findings, and critical incident analysis may highlight performance gaps. Planned changes in procedures, policies, equipment, job descriptions, or care standards suggest anticipated or future learning needs.

FIGURE 11-1 *Formal Learning Needs Assessment Tool*

EMERGENCY DEPARTMENT (ED): EDUCATION NEEDS ASSESSMENT

Years of ED nursing experience: < 1 year; 1–2 years; 3–5 years; 6–10 years; 11–15 years; 16–20 years; > 20 years

Please read each item and circle the number corresponding to your comfort with the equipment:

(5 = Extremely comfortable, 4 = Very comfortable, 3 = Slightly comfortable, 2 = Uncomfortable, 1 = Very uncomfortable)

Arterial line setup	5	4	3	2	1
Autotransfusion	5	4	3	2	1
Cardioversion/defibrillation	5	4	3	2	1
Chest tube drainage setup	5	4	3	2	1
Diagnostic peritoneal lavage	5	4	3	2	1
End-tidal CO_2 monitor	5	4	3	2	1
External pacing	5	4	3	2	1
External ventricular drain setup	5	4	3	2	1
Level I fluid warmer	5	4	3	2	1
Life-Pak 12: AED functions	5	4	3	2	1
Radiant warmer bed (Ohio bed)	5	4	3	2	1
Stryker® Wedge® Turning Frame	5	4	3	2	1
Transvenous pacing	5	4	3	2	1
Venous access devices	5	4	3	2	1

Are there any other procedures/pieces of equipment you would like to review?

What types of patients do you feel *least* comfortable caring for?

List two topics that you would like to learn more about in the coming year.

1.

2.

Adapted from Mager, R.F., & Pipe, P. (1984). *Analyzing performance problems* (2nd ed.). Belmont, CA: Lake Publishing Company.

Diagnosing or Analyzing the Data

Performance is a dynamic interplay between technical skills, interpersonal skills, and critical thinking. Although education is commonly viewed as the primary strategy responsible for improving individual or group performance, instruction may or may not be the most appropriate intervention. Once a need has been identified, the cause(s) of the performance gap should be analyzed. Does the discrepancy exist because of lack of skills or knowledge, lack of incentives or rewards, lack of motivation, inadequate flow of information, or inadequate support systems? Determining the root cause of a performance gap is critical to solving the problem because different causes respond to different interventions. Mager and Pipe[2] developed an algorithm to analyze performance discrepancies as an aid to identifying optimal solutions (Figure 11-2).

FIGURE 11-2 *Analyzing Performance Problems*

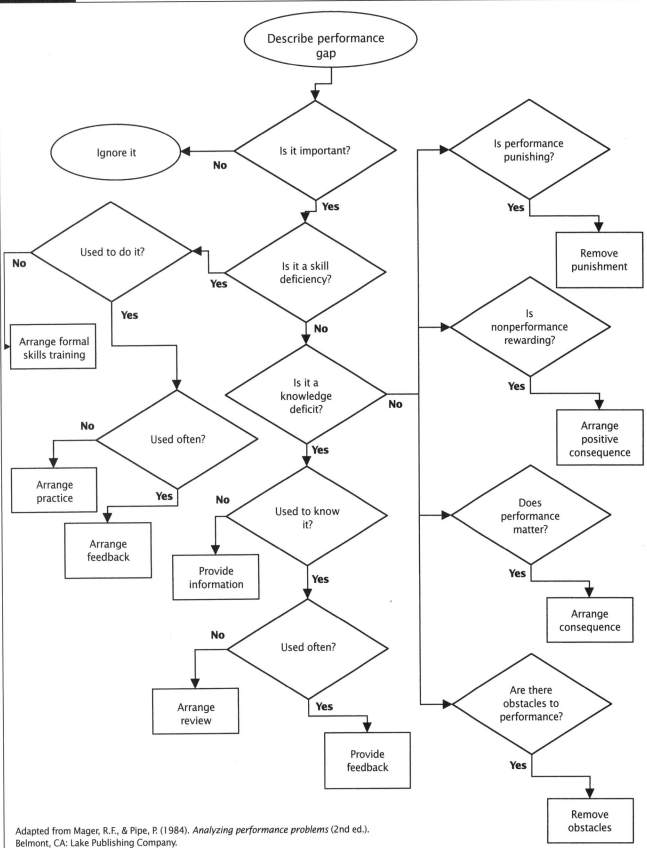

Adapted from Mager, R.F., & Pipe, P. (1984). *Analyzing performance problems* (2nd ed.).
Belmont, CA: Lake Publishing Company.

The left side of the chart addresses performance problems related to knowledge or skill deficiencies (i.e., learning needs), whereas the right-hand side of the chart addresses performance discrepancies related to management of the work environment and functioning in the real world (i.e., nonlearning needs).

Planning the Educational Initiative

Goals and Objectives

Once a learning need has been identified as the root cause of a performance gap, educational planning begins. The first priority is to determine the instructional goal (i.e., What do you want learners to be able to do when they have completed the instruction?). The goal then needs to be analyzed and a step-by-step determination made of what people are doing when they perform the goal and what entry behaviors are needed. Robert Gagne[3] suggests that in designing programs, skills and concepts should be learned one at a time, and lower level objectives must be mastered before higher level objectives can be met (sequenced instruction). His theory stipulates that there are five categories of learning, and each type requires different teaching strategies.

- Motor skills: Precise, smooth and accurately timed execution of performances involving the use of muscles. Instructional strategy: Have learner observe a piece of the task being performed, practice the subtask, receive feedback, and continue to practice the subtask until the subtask can be performed to some degree of mastery; then add the next subtask.

- Verbal information: Declarative knowledge. Instructional strategy: State facts, concepts, or principles orally (e.g., discussions, lectures) or in writing (e.g., independent study).

- Intellectual skills: Discriminations, concepts, or rules. Instructional strategy: Provide opportunities for labeling or classifying, applying rules, demonstrating principles, and problem solving.

- Attitudes: Acquired internal states that influence choices of personal action. Instructional strategy: Associate desired attitude with a credible role model or persuasive arguments using discussion, role play, or simulations.

- Cognitive strategies: Consciously applied techniques for recalling information. Instructional strategy: Devise mnemonics or memory aids.

The performance objectives developed for the program should include: (1) the specific behavioral skills to be learned, (2) the conditions under which they must be performed, and (3) the criteria for successful performance. Objectives include all of the important outcomes of the educational initiative, are in harmony with sound principles of learning, and should be realistic in terms of the abilities of the learner, time, and facilities available.[4] The content of the instruction becomes the information or training the learner needs to master each objective.

Target Audience

Characteristics of the learners (i.e., the target audience) should be considered in designing the teaching strategy. The previous knowledge, experience, and attitudes of the target group toward the content area, their motivation for learning the content, their education and ability levels, and their learning preferences are vital pieces of information for effective planning. Malcolm Knowles[5] described these attributes of adult learners:

- Self-concept: The adult learner is independent and self-directed and appreciates rationale for the existence of the learning experience (i.e., Why do I need/want to know this?). It is a mistake to assume that novice staff members or patients with a new diagnosis can verbalize or direct their learning needs—they simply do not know what they do not know!

- Experience: The adult learner has past experiences in life that enable adaptation to new information (i.e., How does this new information apply to what I already know?).

- Readiness to learn: The adult learner expects and appreciates learning that is immediately applicable to his or her present situation (i.e., How can I use this information in my current circumstances?).

- Orientation to learning: Adults learn best from education that is problem centered (i.e., How is this information going to help me with a problem I'm experiencing?).

- Motivation to learn: Adults have extrinsic and intrinsic motivators for learning (i.e., What will learning this information do for me?). Intrinsic motivators can be very powerful. There are often influential disincentives to learning and adapting new behaviors that need to be recognized and confronted.

Time Frame

A realistic estimate of the amount of time required to design and present the educational initiative should be based on the objectives and subtasks that need to be achieved to meet the overall goal. Multiple factors[6] need to be considered when determining the time allotted for instruction (Table 11-1).

It is preferable to simplify the goal and allow the mastery of a smaller amount of content than to allow insufficient time and incomplete mastery of all the objectives.

Selecting a Teaching Strategy

With the goal(s), objectives, content, type of learning, and target audience defined, an appropriate teaching strategy should be selected. The most effective format will match learning activities with the learning objectives, keeping the learner involved at all times. Teaching strategies should test the learner's new abilities, building success and reinforcement into the instruction. The teacher should make learning fun and allow adequate time to practice skills, incorporating multiple methods of instruction to help build these

Table 11-1
Factors Influencing the Instructional Time Frame
Total time available for instruction
Total number of objectives
Priority assigned to each objective
Nature and complexity of the objectives and subject matter
Learners' present knowledge, skills, attitudes, and experience related to the objectives
Types of teaching strategies to be used
Availability of resources (facilities, personnel, equipment)
Presenter's experience in teaching the subject matter

Table 11-2	
Effect of Teaching Strategies on Content Retention	
STRATEGY	MATERIAL RETAINED
Reading	10%
Listening	20%
Seeing and observing	30%
Listening and observing	50%
Listening, observing, and discussing	70%
Listening, observing, discussing, and performing	90%

skills.[7] Although each person has a learning preference, which is their primary and most comfortable style of learning (i.e., visual, auditory, or kinesthetic), combining a variety of teaching and learning strategies that appeal to multiple senses[8] increases retention (Table 11-2).

Commonly used learning activities include the following.

- Printed materials: Fact sheets, pamphlets, newsletters. This strategy is effective for disseminating essential truths to multiple individuals at multiple points in time. Educators frequently use written materials to convey information to their staff regarding departmental or institutional updates, new medications, and new programs. The majority of patient educational resources (e.g., discharge instructions) are provided in this format. Printed materials can be used to reinforce verbal instruction, but when they are used as the only teaching strategy, it is difficult to determine the learner's understanding of the content or whether the information was actually read. Although patient education materials have been targeted to as low as fourth-grade reading levels, health literacy, or the ability to read, understand, and act on health information, is a growing concern. The American Medical Association estimates that low health literacy adversely affects approximately 90 million Americans and is largely unrecognized by health care providers.[9] Low health literacy affects all ethnic groups, with the greatest prevalence among native-born whites, and is particularly common among the older population and low-income people.
- Group discussions/in-services: Short sessions, generally less than 30 minutes in length; often

directed by specific questions or patient-care issues or used to explain new procedures. This interactive strategy is effective for exchanging verbal information and problem solving. Discussions are often extemporaneous; in-services require the scheduling of repeated sessions if each individual who needs the information is to receive the information.

■ Classes, lectures, seminars, conferences, workshops: Oral presentations of instruction in a prescribed time frame, generally more than 50 minutes. This strategy allows information to be presented to a large group with sufficient time generally allotted for the mastery of multiple objectives and goal(s). This format is most effective in teaching intellectual skills and cognitive behaviors. Participants must be off duty for the scheduled time, which requires scheduling repeated sessions or videotaping if the majority of the staff is to receive the information.

■ Demonstrations: Learner observes desired performance and practices the skill in a return demonstration. This format is highly interactive and effective in teaching psychomotor skills, standards for performance, and interactive skills. Demonstrations require scheduling repeated sessions.

■ Role play: Learners act out their own situation or that of another person. Role reversal is useful for sensitizing one person to the other's situation. This is an effective strategy for learning new attitudes and intellectual skills.

■ Self-directed or programmed instruction: Computer-assisted instruction (CAI), CD-ROMs, books, pamphlets, videotapes, and independent study modules. These strategies are generally formatted to include: (1) the overall purpose of the learning activity, (2) behavioral objectives, (3) learning resources contained within the module, (4) directions for use of the module, (4) a pretest, (5) exercises with feedback that provide for the application of knowledge throughout the module, and (6) a posttest with feedback to measure mastery of the content.[10] This teaching strategy allows core information to be relayed to multiple individuals at multiple points in time, but because it is self-paced, there is often minimal or no interaction with the learner. Both CAI and videotapes require access to the corresponding audiovisual

media. High-quality, commercially produced instructional programs are available for both patient education and clinical topics.

■ Posters: Graphic display of information (e.g., new processes, procedures, or equipment). This format is portable, generally requires minimal space, is reusable, is inexpensive, and allows core information to be relayed to multiple individuals at multiple points in time. There may be minimal interaction with the learner, and it is difficult to ensure that each individual who needs the information reviews the poster.

■ Educational bulletin boards: Graphic display of information, generally larger than a poster; often dedicated to a particular topic (e.g., summer emergencies). This format allows core information to be relayed to multiple individuals at multiple points in time and is most effective for conveying facts. There is minimal interaction for the learner, and it is difficult to determine whether individuals who need the information reviewed it.

■ Case studies: Review of a particular patient case or patient care issue. This strategy is highly interactive and encourages critical thinking. In some institutions, case studies may be presented in an interdisciplinary format (i.e., grand round), allowing the exchange of ideas among the many providers engaged in the patient's care; requires scheduling of repeated sessions if majority of staff are to receive the information.

■ Journal clubs: Discussion of peer-reviewed article(s) on a particular topic. This strategy is highly interactive, promotes critical thinking, and allows participants to examine their current practice in light of research findings, encouraging incorporation of research into practice. In some institutions, the physician and nursing staff may participate in joint journal clubs. Participants must be off duty for the scheduled time; the same topic is rarely repeated.

■ Simulation: Actual reenactment of a real-life situation. This format is highly interactive, encourages critical thinking, and is very effective in teaching psychomotor skills. This strategy is resource intensive and requires scheduling repeated sessions if the majority of staff is to participate.

- Games: Allows participants to learn and/or review concepts in a "fun," nontraditional format (e.g., Jeopardy!® game). Although this promotes enjoyment and interaction, participants may become overly competitive. This format is time consuming to design and requires scheduling repeated sessions if the majority of the staff is to participate.

Implementing the Educational Initiative

Success in the delivery of instruction is based on the presenter's knowledge of the subject matter and communication skills. All necessary materials and supplies (e.g., handouts, audiovisual equipment) should be available before instruction begins. Learning requires four critical elements: (1) motivation, (2) reinforcement, (3) retention, and (4) transfer. A learner must be motivated to learn before any learning takes place (i.e., they must perceive a need to know). Learners must receive some encouragement or reward (i.e., a sense of progress or success) if learning is to continue. This requires feedback between the learner and educator. To benefit from a learning activity, participants must retain the learned knowledge or skills. Retention is directly affected by the opportunity to practice using the new information. Finally, the learner needs to transfer the materials learned to the situation. Gagne[11] states there are nine events that activate the processes needed for learning and believes that all instruction should include this sequence of events (Table 11-3).

Evaluating the Educational Initiative

Evaluation is the process of determining the value and effectiveness of a teaching strategy or program. Kirkpatrick's Four Level Evaluation Model[12] has been universally adopted by the training profession as the framework for evaluating teaching strategies.[13]

- Level 1— Reaction: Evaluation at this level measures how those who participate in a program react to it. It attempts to answer questions regarding the participants' perceptions (e.g., Did they like it? Were the topics completely covered? Was the material relevant to

Table 11-3
The Nine Events of Instruction
1. Gain attention: Draw the learner to the learning.
2. Describe the goal: Explain what the learners will be able to accomplish and how they will be able to use the knowledge.
3. Stimulate recall of prior knowledge: Remind learners of things they already know that are relevant to the current lesson.
4. Present the material to be learned: Teach the skill one subtask at a time.
5. Provide guidance for learning: Give learners some instructions about how to learn it.
6. Elicit performance: Let learners practice the skill or apply the knowledge.
7. Provide informative feedback: Give rationale why performance was correct/incorrect.
8. Assess performance: Test to see whether the lesson has been learned.
9. Enhance retention and transfer to other contexts: Show learners how to apply the lesson/skills/knowledge to real situations they encounter.

their situation/work environment?). Minimally, every teaching strategy or program should be evaluated at this level to provide feedback for improving the methods. Although a positive reaction does not guarantee learning, a negative reaction almost certainly reduces its possibility.

- Level 2—Learning: Evaluation at this level moves beyond learner satisfaction and attempts to assess the extent participants have advanced in skills, knowledge, or attitude as a result of the teaching (i.e., Did they learn anything?). This is commonly measured using self-assessment or a pretest/posttest method. Level 2 evaluation may indicate that teaching strategies are effective or ineffective, but does not prove if newly acquired knowledge or skills will be used.

- Level 3—Transfer: This level of evaluation measures the extent to which a change in behavior has occurred because of the instruction (i.e., Is the newly acquired knowledge, skill, or attitude being applied in the everyday environment of the learner?). Level 3 evaluations often require direct observation (e.g., performance checklist) or formal testing after the learner has completed the education. Behavioral data provide insight into the transfer of information from the teaching setting to the real-life surroundings and the barriers encountered when attempting to incorporate new practices.

- Level 4—Results: This level measures the overall success of the training (e.g., Did it matter? Is it adding value for the organization or patient?). These effects can include such indicators as improved efficiency, patient outcomes, and patient satisfaction, as well as morale and teamwork. Evaluation at this higher level may require gathering additional data or monitoring data already being collected. Evaluation becomes more difficult and time consuming moving from Level 1 to Level 4, but the information is of increasingly significant value to the organization.

Continuing Education Contact Hours

Continuing education is currently required of registered nurses for license renewal in 26 states; 31 states require continuing education for APNs.[14] Specialty certification (e.g., Certified Emergency Nurse and Certified Critical Care Registered Nurse) requires a specified numbers of contact hours for recertification via contact hours. Many institutions have been granted Provider Approval status by their states' nurses' association/American Nurses Credentialing Center Commission on Accreditation and have an internal review process for awarding contact hours. Contact hours for programs may also be awarded by specialty organizations, such as Emergency Nurses Association or American Association of Colleges of Nursing.

The APN should consider applying for contact hours for all eligible educational initiatives. Knowing that contact hours are awarded may encourage attendance at programs and may encourage staff members to sit for specialty certification because many of the contact hours required for recertification are available on-site.

Summary

The APN is strategically positioned to facilitate both formal and informal learning. Education of patients and the community is vital for maintaining and preserving health. The continuing education of emergency nursing staff "promotes competence in nursing, enhances nurse's working knowledge, advances skills in education, research, administration, and theory development, improves health care in the client, and fosters personal and professional development as well as career goals"[15] so that quality patient care can be sustained and advanced. The effectiveness of the APN in creating meaningful learning opportunities is enhanced through applying the components of the nursing process to the development of educational initiatives.

REFERENCES

1. Burton, J. K., & Merrill, P. F. (1991). Needs assessment: Goals, needs, and priorities. In L. J. Briggs, K. L. Gustafson, & M. H. Tillman (Eds.), *Instructional design: Principles and applications* (2nd ed., pp. 17–43). Englewood Cliffs, NJ: Educational Technology Publications.
2. Mager, R. F., & Pipe, P. (1984). *Analyzing performance problems* (2nd ed.). Belmont, CA: Lake Publishing Company.
3. Gagne, R. (1985). *The conditions of learning* (4th ed.). New York: Holt, Rinehart & Winston.
4. Gronlund, N. E. (1995). *How to write and use instructional objectives* (5th ed.). Englewood Cliffs, NJ: Prentice Hall.
5. Knowles, M. S., Holton, E. F., III, & Swanson, K. A. (1998). *The adult learner: The definitive classic in adult education and human resource development* (5th ed.). Houston, TX: Gulf Publishing.
6. Alspach, J. G. (1995). *The educational process in nursing staff development.* St. Louis, MO: Mosby.
7. Rankin, S. H., & Stallings, K. D. (1996). *Patient education, issues, principles, practice* (3rd ed., p. 195). Philadelphia: Lippincott-Raven.
8. Weinland, J. D. (1957). *How to improve your memory.* New York: Harper & Row.
9. *Facts About Health Literacy.* (2002, April 16). Retrieved April 30, 2002 from http://www.ama-assn.org/ama/pub/category/7805.html
10. Gianella, A. (1996). Effective teaching and learning strategies for adults. In R. S. Abruzzese (Ed.), *Nursing staff development: Strategies for success* (2nd ed., pp. 227–228). St. Louis, MO: Mosby.
11. Gagne, R., Briggs, L., & Wager, W. (1992). *Principles of instructional design* (4th ed.). Fort Worth, TX: HBJ College Publishers.
12. Kirkpatrick, D. (1994). *Evaluating training programs.* San Francisco: Berrett-Koehler.
13. Hale, J. (2000, September/October). Applying Kirkpatrick's four levels of evaluation. *Training Today,* 9–12.
14. *ANA/ANF launch new continuing education web site for RNs.* (1999, May 6). Retrieved April 30, 2002 from http://nursingworld.org/pressrel/1999/pr0506.htm
15. Bracken, L. J., & Martinez, R. R. (2000). Education. In K. S. Jordan (Ed.), *Emergency nursing core curriculum* (5th ed., pp. 751–764). Philadelphia: Saunders.

12 LIFESTYLE BEHAVIOR CHANGE: MOVING FROM HEALTH-RISKING TO HEALTH-PROMOTING BEHAVIORS

Barbara W. Bollenberg, RN, PhD(c), CEN

Emergency nursing clinicians care for patients with health-risking behaviors on a daily basis. This group of patients may arguably pose one of the greatest quandaries in emergency nursing practice. Although we are used to multitasking, when it comes to facilitating change among patients or staff, most advanced practice nurses (APNs) are at a loss to know how to begin the process. There is a confusing and broad array of advice. What are the best techniques to promote change in our relatively brief encounters with these patients? We are positioned to care for patients during their most vulnerable moments. We have an opportunity to move patients in the direction of positive change. It is our challenge to accomplish this while tending to the conflicting priorities of the emergency department (ED) and finding the most expeditious way to meet our patient's change needs. This chapter will give the APN better knowledge and understanding of the behavior change process. The APN will also find specific tools to facilitate positive behavioral change for the ED patient population.

Inpatient settings usually provide hours if not days for nursing staff to work with behavioral change of patients. The nature of the ED visit means that the nurse will have a relatively brief amount of time to help the patient identify and work on change goals. This chapter will help the APN focus on meeting the change needs of emergency patients. Health-risking behaviors contribute to many of the illnesses and injuries that are treated by emergency clinicians. Prochaska illustrated the scope of the problem when he said that approximately half the cost of health care is directly related to health-risking behaviors.[1] This is particularly visible in the ED in which we see patients who smoke, drink, abuse other substances, overeat, fail to exercise or to wear their seat belts,

do not take their medications as prescribed, and in general abuse their bodies and test their luck. These patients sometimes become our "frequent flyers." These are the patients that we see time and time again, often for the same precipitating factors. One ED registered nurse (RN) repeatedly counseled a chronic obstructive pulmonary disease patient about the critical importance of smoking cessation. On one occasion when he returned to the ED with an exacerbation of his emphysema, he emphatically declared that he had taken the RN's advice to quit smoking. When she helped him get dressed after treatment, a pack of cigarettes and a lighter fell out of his pants. He looked at the nurse straight-faced and said, "I'm keeping these for a friend." In an ideal world, the nurse and the patient would identify a problem and develop change goals, and the patient would make the desired change. In the real world there are conflicting priorities and barriers to change that test both the nurse's skills and the patient's resolve.

In addition to the change needs of patients, clinicians often have change issues of their own. How seriously do patients take the advice of a nurse with smoke on her breath or from a physician who is morbidly obese? There is clear convincing evidence that a healthy diet that is lower in fat and portion controlled plus regular exercise are important to long-term health. It is difficult to consider fat-free cottage cheese when the break room is supplied with doughnuts. It is hard to find energy for regular exercise when you've just finished a killer shift and can barely move. The demands of a busy and involved life make it hard to find time for health-promoting behaviors. Many of us also have spouses or other family members who have health-risking behaviors and look to us for advice. What has been done to find answers to behavior change questions? This chapter explores the lifestyle behavior change phenomena and samples some of the seminal theories that have been the foundation for our current understanding of behavior change. There are also guidelines and strategies for treating patients with varying levels of readiness to change and tools to use to identify how ready your patient is to change a problem behavior.

Overview of Lifestyle Behavior Change Theories and Models

Health care educators and clinicians have long sought the answers to health behavior problems. What is the most effective way to move patients from health-risking to health-promoting behaviors? At present there are over 400 theories that attempt to find solutions to this problem. Some theories focus on a single tenet. Other theories and models attack change in a more complex and comprehensive way. Reviewing the best-known and most studied change theories will illustrate how change science has evolved to its current level. One of the classic change theorists is Kurt Lewin.[2,3] Lewin's early work with Swiss schoolchildren led to his foundational Field Theory, which is the basis for many current health education programs. Lewin was considered a cognitive theorist who emphasized the value that an individual places on an outcome and focused on the individual's belief that a given action would result in the desired outcome. The association between the individual's perception of the outcome and the ability to achieve that outcome has been described in this context as value expectancy theory. Lewin is also credited as the father of stage theory.[3] The first stage begins with the unfreezing of an undesirable behavior or attitude. The second stage exposes the individual to new (desirable) information, perspectives, and theory. It is hoped that the individual adopts the new behavior, and then in the third stage the clinician works to maintain or freeze the new behavior pattern through reinforcement and support. Lewin's theory is recognized not only for its contribution to individual therapy, but also for its reputation as the model for most organizational change theories.

Skinner[3] was one of the human behavior change pioneers. He is credited with the concept of oper-

ant conditioning in which behavior is influenced by knowledge of the consequences of the act. The behavior must be voluntary, and subjects must be clearly aware of the cause-and-effect relationship of their actions to the outcome. For example, a child who touches a hot stove and is burned learns not to repeat the action for fear of being burned again.

Stuart[4] identified operant conditioning techniques that have been used to reduce undesirable behaviors. For example, when an individual is punished each time he or she repeats a behavior, this serves as a deterrent to repetition of the behavior. An example of this might be a parental decision to take away a teenager's driving privileges after a missed curfew. Another operant conditioning technique used to decrease behaviors is extinction (the process of eliminating the undesirable behavior by ignoring the behavior or removing any reward or recognition connected to the behavior). This decreases the probability that the behavior will recur. When young children act out to get attention from a parent, the parent may be instructed to ignore the behavior, only providing attention when the child acts within acceptable limits.

Another form of operant conditioning is positive reinforcement. Positive reinforcement rewards the individual whenever the desired behavior is performed. When the behavior is associated with an expected reward, the behavior is more likely to be repeated. Using positive reward, a smoker may choose to use the money not spent on cigarettes to save for a special trip or a gift. As an alternative, the therapist may utilize negative reinforcement (such as aversive therapy). In this case, the subject avoids the aversive stimuli by performing the desirable behavior. This is negative reinforcement, but it is also likely to have the desired effect on behavioral outcome. This author's husband quit smoking in a program that delivered mild electric shocks while he smoked in a smoke-filled booth. This successful effort linked the aversive stimulus with the smoking behavior.

Aversive therapy is not clinically practical for the ED and is not in sync with the positive proactive image of the emergency clinician. How, then, do we move our patients in the direction of change? Miller and Rolnick[5] suggest that motivation is the key to redirecting lifestyle behaviors. A key strategy is motivational interviewing. Although this technique was first used with alcoholics, it is useful when working with anyone who needs to make a behavior change. There are five general principles that form the motivational interviewing approach: (1) express empathy ("It must be very hard to think about quitting smoking when you have been doing it for 30 years."); (2) develop discrepancy ("You say that your health is important to you. How can you say that and keep smoking?"); (3) avoid argumentation (Don't put the patient in a position of arguing in favor of the unhealthy behavior while you argue against it.); (4) roll with resistance (change tactics, redirect, distract); and (5) support self-efficacy (The individual's belief that he or she has the ability to perform the behavior necessary to achieve a desired outcome; "You know you can do this.").

Warm personal interactions that use reflection, open-ended questions, and a nonjudgmental style facilitate the counseling process. The patient is taught that some ambivalence is expected. The clinician offers support to strengthen the patient's desire for change. The patient develops discrepancy when comparing personal health goals with the behavior that is detrimental to those goals. The clinician avoids arguing with the patient (no matter how faulty the patient's reasoning might be). When resistance is met, it is a cue to reevaluate treatment strategy and to consider another approach. The clinician supports self-efficacy by helping the patient to recognize and build on both strengths and successes. It is stressed that the individual has the power to make the change; the clinician or others do not impose change. Motivational interviewing provides specific guidelines for intervening with the majority of patients who are not yet ready for change. A relative drawback to this approach is the amount of time (45 to 120 minutes) that Miller and Rolnick recommend for each intervention. In emergency nursing practice, it would be rare to have this amount of time to counsel patients.

Another well-known change theory is the Health Belief Model[6] (HBM). In the early 1950s there was an outbreak of tuberculosis. The U.S. Public Health Service thought that by offering free chest x-rays, they would identify cases and institute early treatment. Unfortunately, this idea was a dismal failure; few people took advantage of the free x-ray offer. The HBM resulted when social psychologists sought to explain this lack of success and to identify factors that would either inhibit or facilitate public participation in health initiatives. This model is considered a value expectancy theory (meaning that the individual weighs the value of avoiding illness or regaining health against the belief that health-promoting behaviors could have a positive effect on illness avoidance or health improvement). The individual further evaluates his or her own perceived susceptibility to illness or injury and the likelihood that the individual's actions would directly affect health outcomes.

The HBM as presently stated has several components.[6,7] These include perceived susceptibility (subjective understanding of personal risk), perceived severity (the degree of threat perceived by the individual, i.e., death, disability, or pain), and perceived benefit (positive effects on health outcomes). Further, the HBM also identified possible barriers to action, such as difficulty, perceptions of expense, or inconvenience. An important subconcept of the HBM is cues to action. Some early HBM research suggested that readiness to change might be facilitated by cues to take action. These cues would vary with the individual. A cue might be as subtle as a glance in the mirror revealing the need to lose weight and start exercise or as obvious as a smoker whose spouse is found to have lung cancer. Socioeconomic factors such as environment, income, and education are also thought to affect health beliefs. Self-efficacy, or the individual's belief that he or she can achieve the health-promoting goals necessary to achieve the desired outcome, is the final component of the HBM.

Clark and Becker describe the HBM as encompassing both the personal value that individuals place on a specific goal and individuals' expectations that their actions can achieve that goal.[7] They describe the model as most appropriate for health-related behaviors that are associated with attitudes and beliefs. The model is also based on the premise that health is the ultimate goal for most individuals. In contrast, some individuals may diet (even to an excessive degree) solely for appearance sake or be unable to change a health-risking occupation for economic reasons. When health is not the individual's goal, or when the usual cues to action are not present, the HBM is not helpful in explaining behavior.

Bandura[8,9] introduced the Social Cognitive Theory (SCT), which acknowledges both the inter- and intrapersonal factors that influence behavior and promote behavioral change. One construct of the SCT is reciprocal determinism. This construct identifies the interaction between an individual's personal characteristics, behavior, and environment. A change in one dimension is reflected by change in the other two dimensions. Other constructs of the SCT include environmental (external factors that influence behavior), learning while watching others, and behavioral capability (knowledge and skill required to accomplish the desired behavior). Reinforcement rewards the individual for the desired behavior and increases the likelihood of the repetition of the behavior. The individual learns outcome expectations (the belief that certain outcomes occur in response to particular behaviors) and develops outcome expectancies that weigh the value of the outcome to the person. Self-efficacy is also important in SCT. The individual must have confidence in the ability to perform a desired behavior despite perceived barriers.

The Theory of Reasoned Action (TRA) and the Theory of Planned Behavior (TPB) models both focus on the individual's motivation to change behavior. Fishbein[10] introduced the TRA in an effort to explain the link between attitudes and behavior. A person who highly values a behavior outcome is more likely to repeat the behavior. If the behavior is associated with a negative outcome, a person is less likely to repeat the behavior. The TPB builds on the TRA and the work of Ajzen and Fishbein.[11] It adds the idea of the individual's perception of the ability to manipulate or control factors that are external to the individual. External factors may be additional barriers to effecting the desired change, or they may facilitate the behavior change. For example, a change in job smoking rules could make it easier for an individual to decide to quit smoking.

Cox[12] is a nurse who developed an interaction model of client health behavior. Her model recog-

nizes the client's individuality or uniqueness in seeking healthy behaviors, addresses the influence of client/professional interactions on health behaviors, and recommends nursing interventions tailored specifically for the individual and that person's health care needs. Cox felt that many behavior change models were too closely aligned with a particular discipline such as psychology or sociology, which (in her view) limited their effectiveness. She believed that models that cross several domains tend to be more effective with families or communities instead of facilitating individual change. Cox also reminds us that earlier models were developed in different times (when the focus was on disease instead of health promotion). Her third issue with established behavior change models is that they tend to be global and do not provide clear direction for professionals attempting to incorporate them into clinical practice. Cox proposed the use of an Interaction Model of Client Health Behavior, which presupposes the client's ability to make informed health care decisions. Cox's model lets the clinician assume the role of teacher/guide (not decision maker). Cox recognizes the singularity (individuality) of each person (a unique combination of background, motivation, health concerns, and personal responses) that is the primary determinant of the behavior change outcome.

Another important nurse behavior change theorist is Pender,[13] who discusses "modifications" of health-related lifestyle and describes her Health Promotion Model (HPM) as an approach-oriented model. She sees this as more useful in motivating healthy lifestyles than previous negative avoidance models. Pender described her model as "an attempt to depict the multidimensional nature of persons interacting with their environment as they pursue health."[13] The HPM uses features from both the HBM and SCT within a nursing framework of "holistic human functioning."[13]

Prochaska and DiClemente[14] proposed a Transtheoretical Model (TTM) that crossed several theories to explain how people change behavior. Prochaska, Norcross, and DiClemente[15] studied the "why" and "how" of successful self-changers and found distinctive patterns of readiness to change. Prochaska, working with DiClemente, found that individuals could be

Table 12-1	
Stages of Change	
Precontemplation	The stage in which people have no intention of changing behavior and typically deny having a problem
Contemplation	The stage in which people acknowledge that they have a problem and think seriously about changing it
Preparation	The stage in which people are planning to take action within the next month and are making the final adjustments before they begin to change their behavior
Action	The stage in which people most overtly modify their behavior and their surroundings. They make the change for which they've been preparing
Maintenance	The stage in which people work to consolidate the gains attained during the action and previous stages and struggle to prevent lapse or relapse

grouped into stages of change dependent on readiness to actualize the change. Prochaska and DiClemente[16] define these stages as shown in Table 12-1.

It has been suggested that the terms *precontemplation* and *contemplation* are somewhat stilted and awkward to use. Instead of precontemplation, this author uses the term *unconcerned*. These are patients who may or may not recognize that their health-risking behaviors are unhealthy, but don't view the behavior as a real problem. Often these patients will say, "If you have to die from something, it might as well be something you like." In contrast, the patient in the stage that Prochaska and DiClemente[16] call contemplation could more accurately be described as "considering." These patients are aware that their habit poses a risk or problem for them, and they are weighing the pros and cons of the behavior with the pros and cons of quitting.

Prochaska and DiClemente[16] also created a short-form assessment tool to assist self-changers in identifying their stage of change. By answering four short questions, the self-changer can distinguish which stage of change he or she is in and take action appropriately. The TTM short-form assessment tool is as follows.[16]

1. I solved my problem more than six months ago.
2. I have taken action on my problem within the past six months.
3. I am intending to take action in the next month.

4. I am intending to take action in the next six months.

Someone who answers "No" to each of these statements is in the precontemplation stage. Someone who answers "Yes" to question one is in the maintenance stage of change. Someone who answers "Yes" to question two is in the action stage of change. Someone who answers "Yes" to questions three and four would be in the preparation stage. This short form can be used to identify patients' readiness to change so that we can plan appropriate strategies to meet their needs.

In an even simpler way to gauge readiness to change, this author sometimes draws a horizontal line (about three inches long) on a piece of paper and marks one end "ready to change" and the other end "not ready to change." Then the patient is asked to put an X on the line to correspond with feelings of being ready to make the change being discussed with the clinician. This is an easy visual way for both the patient and clinician to assess readiness to change.

Identifying the Most Effective Strategies for Lifestyle Behavior Change

The idea of meeting the patient at his or her stage of readiness and tailoring change strategies to the individual needs is consistent with the patient-centered approach of nursing. The Stages of Change and the TTM are one of the most important developments in meeting the change needs of all patients, not just the limited few who present to the ED ready to change health-risking behaviors. However, the TTM (as discussed previously) doesn't directly address all change needs of the widely diverse ED population. There is still a need to explore how patients change and to develop strategies that are effective in the fast-paced ED setting. Using the TTM as inspiration this author developed a Change Synthesis Model (CHASM) to explain how individuals change health care behaviors. This model focuses on the opportunity to facilitate change for every patient (not just the limited number who are actually ready to change). Table 12-2 outlines strategies that have come from this model.

Knowing patients' readiness to change is critical to guiding them toward effective change processes. Clinicians seeking to facilitate change must also utilize individualized strategies to move the patient from health-risking to health-promoting behaviors. The author has studied subjects who successfully changed a health-risking behavior (stopped smoking) to see if these individuals changed in ways that are consistent with the CHASM model. For example one of the variables included in CHASM is the concept of a trigger or cue that facilitates change (in this case, smoking cessation). Early study results do indicate that a trigger such as bad health news or pressure from family members or friends is important in facilitating change. Although the literature has long supported clear unequivocal language in telling patients to quit smoking,[17] several pilot test subjects reported that their clinician's words were particularly effective for them. One was told, "You can breathe or you can smoke, it's your choice." Another subject had a painful vascular procedure done after her doctor linked her condition to years of smoking. She quit smoking on the spot declaring, "I was never going to let them hurt me like that again." Another subject who had survived coronary bypass surgery and lung cancer was not moved to quit smoking until his grandchildren convinced him that they needed him "to be around." That interaction compelled him to quit after 50 plus years of smoking.

One key component of CHASM is individualism. For example, if we put 20 emergency nurses in one room and told them that they needed to lose 10 pounds, we would expect to see 20 different approaches to the problem. Some nurses might increase exercise while modifying their diets, whereas some might rely solely on diet or exercise alone. Some might head to Subway®, whereas others might consider Slim-Fast®. Some nurses might rely on the Zone or Atkins diet, and some might consider some promising "miracle diet" product they saw on a late-night infomercial. It is also a sure bet that despite any evidence to the contrary, some of the nurses would deny that they had a problem with weight and would simply chose to ignore it. In the future, we may have change boutiques or change smorgasbords in which clients will be able to choose from various change options and strategies. At present, it is important to recognize the individuality of the person we are treating and to offer strategies that are appropriate to that person's readiness to make the change.

Table 12-2
Strategies to Facilitate Change Related to CHASM

1. Assess readiness for change. Focus on cues promoting change.
2. Assist patient in identifying personal health-related values (family, autonomy, health, etc.)
3. Facilitate recognition of personal risk from the behavior. Provide objective evidence. For example, when facilitating smoking cessation, show the patient his or her chest x-ray and point out smoking-related changes, show that the SpO_2 is below the norm, point out clubbing of fingertips, or any other negative consequence of smoking.
4. Emphasize positive benefits of the lifestyle change. Tip the cost/benefit balance in favor of the change. Increase awareness of risks from failure to change.
5. Assist the patient in setting priorities, identifying realistic goals, and committing to change.
6. Strengthen self-efficacy for change. Identify past successes (consider halo effect).
7. Help the patient to anticipate barriers and to develop strategies to counter them.
8. Keep the patient focused on the goal. Remind the patient that this is a priority and that the person has control over the behavior (and not the other way around).
9. Encourage patients to identify strong helping relationships (family members, coworkers, and friends).
10. Recognize success. Provide continued encouragement and support.

Table 12-3	
Counseling Strategies	
STAGE[15,16]	STRATEGY

Precontemplation (Unconcerned): Not intending to take action in the foreseeable future	■ Examine client belief system
	■ Identify values: family, health, spirituality
	■ Identify personal reasons for quitting
	■ Develop discrepancy between personal behavior and personal goals
	■ Raise consciousness (observation, confrontation, interpretation)
	  □ Identify conflict: behavior vs. values
	  □ Identify personal risk (Connect symptoms: Morning cough, DOE, CXR changes)
	■ Educate about the risk of cardiac and lung disease, cancer
	  □ Increase awareness that problem exists
	■ Ask smoker to envision life as a nonsmoker
	■ Inform smoker of new research and strategies that facilitate the quit process and increase opportunities for success
	■ Avoid argumentation
	■ Express empathy
	■ Strongly advise smoker to quit

Contemplation (Considering): Intending to change within the next six months	■ Tip the cost/benefit balance
	■ Stress positives of being a nonsmoker
	  □ Improved sense of taste and smell
	  □ Decreased upper respiratory infections
	  □ Decreased risk of cancer, lung, and heart disease
	  □ Increased self esteem/identity as a nonsmoker
	■ Emphasize risks of not changing
	■ Strengthen self-efficacy for change
	■ Reevaluate past quit attempts
	  □ Identify past successes
	  □ Identify potential barriers/suggest strategies to overcome them
	■ Reduce barriers
	■ Consider social unacceptablity of smoking/effect of smoke on others

Preparation: Intending to take action in the immediate future (usually within one month)	■ Recognize signs of reduced resistance and commitment to readiness to change ■ Build positive and accurate expectations about results ■ Aid client in setting change goals ■ Help client determine best course of action (cold turkey, warm chicken, nicotine fading, pharmacological aids, acupuncture, hypnosis, group programs, etc.) ■ Identify barriers/develop strategy/plan ■ Make commitment to change ■ Set quit date ■ Develop contingency plan to use when tempted to smoke ■ Inform family and friends and ask for their support ■ Consider written (behavioral) smoking cessation contract ■ Develop exercise plan (including relaxation exercises) ■ Practice saying: "No thank you, I don't smoke" ■ Encourage self-rewards ■ Continue to strengthen self-efficacy

Action: Made/making overt lifestyle behavior change within the last six months	■ Throw away cigarettes, ashtrays, matches, etc.
	■ Use nicotine replacement/Zyban® as needed
	■ Avoid smoking triggers
	■ Avoid smokers
	■ Avoid smoky places
	■ Enlist support group to
	  □ Share smoke-free activities
	  □ Talk patient through urges
	  □ Give rewards/praise

(continued)

Table 12-3

Counseling Strategies (continued)	
STAGE[15,16]	STRATEGY

Action: Made/making overt lifestyle behavior change within the last six months (continued)	▫ Be tolerant of moods
	▫ Identify positive changes
	▫ Express confidence in ability to remain nonsmoker
	■ Implement exercise plan
	■ Use relaxation techniques (hot bath, massage, stretching)
	■ Avoid coffee, tea, or colas
	■ Drink extra juice and water
	■ Take a daily multivitamin
	■ Consider hypnosis/self-hypnosis
	■ Use smoking alternatives: gum, celery sticks, toothpicks, cinnamon sticks
	■ Snapping a rubber band on the wrist when feeling the urge to smoke
	■ Remind patient to reward him-/herself for successes
	■ Remind patient
	  ▫ Withdrawal is temporary
	  ▫ Urges are short lived
	  ▫ Withdrawal is a sign that the body is healing itself
	■ Change habits associated with smoking
	■ Decrease negatives/increase positives in life[18]
	■ Provide intratreatment support
	■ Consider using four Ds when urge to smoke hits
	  ▫ Delay
	  ▫ Deep breathe
	  ▫ Drink water
	  ▫ Do something to take your mind off smoking[19]
	■ Also consider four As
	  ▫ Avoid places/people where you are tempted to smoke
	  ▫ Alter—switch to water and soft drinks instead of coffee/alcohol
	  ▫ Alternatives—use oral substitutes
	  ▫ Activities that keep hands busy can be distracting[19]
	■ Have clothes and interior of car cleaned
	■ Encourage stress management techniques
	■ Facilitate client's coping skills
	■ Continue follow-up at designated intervals
	■ Prepare for lapses

Maintenance: Working to prevent relapse (for smokers estimated to last from six months to five years)	■ Continue contingency management ■ Continue follow-up at designated intervals ■ Plan anniversary celebration ■ Emphasize benefits of nonsmoking/personal reasons to quit ■ Help patient with relapse prevention strategies
Termination: Stage where there is zero temptation and 100% efficacy	■ Continue follow-up support at every contact ■ Encourage self-monitoring ■ Review coping strategies/alternative responses ■ Practice/rehearse these strategies ■ Continue to monitor temptations

Table 12-3 provides guidelines for the nurse who is counseling a patient who needs to change and offers samples of strategies that have been used successfully to facilitate lifestyle behavior change (smoking cessation, for example). The emergency nurse sees the patient at a time of vulnerability.

The patient's reason for seeking care may be directly related to a health-risking behavior, and this gives the nurse an opportunity to intervene and suggest the need to change. Although only 20% of patients who need to change are thought to be ready to actually make the change at any given time, the nurse can move the patient in the direction of positive change. General guidelines are suggested in Table 12-4 that may facilitate a health-promoting change.

These brief steps take moments to implement and can have a life-altering effect. Meeting the challenge of lifestyle behavior change is a daily concern for the emergency nursing clinician. In our comparatively brief encounters with a seemingly endless stream of patients, we can make a difference by facilitating health-promoting change. By understanding the complex dynamic of change, we know that some clients will go through many cycles of change before a successful outcome. Yet we know that even "frequent flyers" can be "grounded" and have their lives transformed by successful change. Work with your patients to move them in the direction of change and to make a difference in their futures.

Table 12-4

General Guidelines to Facilitate Health-Promoting Change

1. The patient sees the nurse as an advocate and as a clinical expert who has provided care in the ED encounter.
2. The nurse would clarify the patient's personal risk from the behavior by asking if the patient is aware of the effect of the behavior on the body (i.e., change in liver enzymes from alcohol, decrease in SpO_2, x-ray changes, or frequent upper respiratory infections from smoking).
3. Remind patients that the body is telling them that it is time for a change.
4. Give strong unequivocal advice to quit.
5. Offer help/resources as needed. Develop an arsenal of information for dealing with the most common health behavior problems such as obesity, substance abuse, or smoking that you can give the patient to take home and consider.
6. Tell patients that although they may not feel ready now, the change is needed, and they should consider how they could accomplish it.
7. Remind patients that new research and lifestyle strategies make change possible for everyone.

REFERENCES

1. Prochaska, J. (1995). A conversation with James Prochaska. *Medical Interface, 8,* 50–62.
2. Lewin, K. (1935). *A dynamic theory of personality.* New York: McGraw-Hill.
3. Lewin, K. (1951). The nature of field theory. In M. Marx (Ed.), *Psychological theory.* New York: Macmillan.
4. Stuart, G. W. (1995). Cognitive and behavioral therapy. In G. Stuart & S. Sundeen (Eds.), *Principles and practices of psychiatric nursing* (pp. 747–765). St. Louis, MO: Mosby.
5. Miller, W., & Rolnick, S. (1991). *Motivational interviewing: Preparing people to change addictive behavior.* New York: Guilford.
6. Rosenstock, I., Strecher, V., & Becker, M. (1988). Social learning theory and the health belief model. *Health Education Quarterly, 15*(2), 175–183.
7. Clark, N., & Becker, M. (1988). Theoretical models and strategies for improving adherence and disease management. In S. Shumaker, E. Schron, J. Ockene, & W. McBee (Eds.), *The handbook of health behavior change.* New York: Springer.
8. Bandura, A. (1977). *Social learning theory.* Englewood Cliffs, NJ: Prentice Hall.
9. Bandura, A. (1991). Social cognitive theory of self regulation. *Organization Behavior and Human Decision Processes, 50,* 248–285.
10. Fishbein, M. (1967). *Readings in attitude theory and advances in nursing science measurement.* New York: Wiley.
11. Ajzen, L., & Fishbein, M. (1980). *Understanding attitudes and predicting social behavior.* Englewood Cliffs, NJ: Prentice Hall.
12. Cox, C. (1982, October). An interaction model of client health behavior. *Theoretical Prescription for Nursing,* 41–56.
13. Pender, N. (1986). *Health promotion in nursing practice* (3rd ed.). Stamford, CT: Appleton & Lange.
14. Prochaska, J., & DiClemente, C. (1984). *The transtheoretical approach: Crossing the traditional boundaries of therapy.* Malabar, FL: Krieger.
15. Prochaska, J., Norcross, J., & DiClemente, C. (1994). *Changing for good: A revolutionary six-stage program for overcoming bad habits and moving your life positively forward.* New York: Avon.
16. Prochaska, J., & DiClemente, C. (1982). Self-change processes, self-efficacy, and self-concept in relapse and maintenance of cessation of smoking. *Psychological Reports, 51,* 983–990.
17. American Lung Association. (1998). *Freedom from smoking.* New York: Author.
18. Shipley, R. (1997). *Quit smart.* Durham, NC: JB Press.
19. American Cancer Society. (1997). *Smoking cessation manual.* Atlanta, GA: Author.

PRECEPTORSHIP OF ADVANCED PRACTICE GRADUATE STUDENTS

Kathleen Evanovich Zavotsky, MS, RN, CCRN, CNS, C, CEN

Introduction

The advanced practice nurse (APN) can be the most valuable resource for many health care institutions as well as for patients and families.[1] How the APN student is mentored or preceptored can have a major impact on how the role is utilized. The benefits of mentoring an APN student can be rewarding both professionally and personally. This relationship between APNs and their students may lead to a career-long relationship or mentorship. The confident APN demonstrates a high standard of practice that will be a model for the APN student.

This chapter will review how to become a preceptor and educate and evaluate the APN student. Some of the benefits of taking on this challenge will also be discussed.

How to Become a Preceptor for an APN

First and foremost, as an APN you must want to fulfill this important role and realize the responsibility and commitment that go with it. Professional characteristics of a good preceptor are (1) clinical expertise, (2) interest in professional growth and mastery of clinical skills, (3) excellent leadership and communication skills, (4) learner advocacy, and (5) ability to understand available resources. Personal characteristics include patience, enthusiasm, nonjudgmental attitude toward others, flexibility, open-mindedness, and trustworthiness. Preceptoring an APN student may be a stressful experience, so a sense of humor and self-confidence may be useful throughout the semester.[2]

Often the preceptor–student relationship may turn into a lifelong mentor–mentee relationship. Mentorship is an intense, career-building, mutually beneficial relationship between two individuals of unequal power in an organization. Mentors may serve as a source of information and support.[3]

After you have made the professional decision to take on the role, it is important to discuss this with your supervisor to ensure that time will be allotted for you to meet this responsibility. For many APNs, the role of preceptoring graduate students may already be incorporated into their job description, and if it is not, you may want to consider adding it with the next revision. Take the time to explore what you and your organization have to offer that may be appealing to a graduate student. For example, if you are part of a large university hospital that has just recently started a trauma program, this experience may be of interest to a graduate student. The nurse practitioner (NP) student may want to gain clinical experience with resuscitation, and the clinical nurse specialist (CNS) student may be more interested in development of the staff and new policies and procedures related to trauma care.

Next you will want to contact academic colleagues at local universities to promote yourself as an APN who is interested in preceptoring. When you contact the university, ask if they would be willing to share their curriculum to help guide you in your planning. Offer the faculty a tour of the facility, and have data available that adequately describes your emergency department (Table 13-1). Have your curriculum vitae (CV) updated to distribute to the faculty. Your CV should highlight your clinical expertise and teaching and research accomplishments as well as any publications.

Table 13-1

Statistics to Provide University Faculty to Describe Your ED

- Number of patients seen in the ED per year and per day
- Percentage of adult, pediatric, trauma, and other specialties
- Unique procedures that are performed in the ED: arterial lines, pulmonary artery lines, intracranial pressure monitoring
- Specialty services offered: Sexual Assault Nurse Examiner program, transplantation services, interventional cardiology laboratory
- Payor mix
- Resources available: physicians, APNs, social workers, pharmacists, residency program

Reviewing the conceptual model of the university you are interested in working with will help determine if you can work together with the faculty to accomplish the same goals. In meeting with the faculty, it is important to see if there are opportunities for either a joint appointment or a clinical faculty appointment. Some universities offer monetary compensation or an honorarium for preceptoring graduate students. It is important to review this with the hospital administration prior to accepting either of these if the work is being done on hospital time.

According to Larrabee,[4] the most fundamental ingredient for creating a mutually beneficial joint appointment between a school of nursing and a service organization is visionary leaders in both organizations who are willing to develop a relationship that is goal directed. The creation of a joint appointment should capitalize on the strengths or expertise of a particular nurse to help meet the goals. All parties involved, including the appointee, should have an opportunity to evaluate the role to determine if the expected outcomes have been met at a predetermined time.

Once you and the university have made an agreement, the expectations should be written out in the form of a letter of agreement that in most cases is prepared by the university. This letter should be reviewed closely by yourself and your supervisor to ensure that you both agree with the requirements. In addition to the APN signing the form, most universities require the signature of a hospital administrator.

Clinical affiliations can be beneficial to all involved, but proper planning and communication of expectations should be discussed. During the clinical experience the student must adhere to the hospital's policies and procedures as well as to complete any hospital competency or orientation requirement.[5] Many hospitals appoint one individual to manage the clinical affiliations. This individual is often an educator from a nursing education department who is familiar with the regulations.

The university should also provide the hospital with appropriate university policies and procedures that could affect the faculty and/or student. For example, if a student presents to the clinical area impaired by either alcohol or drugs, what should the preceptor do? Spier et al.[6] developed a policy to help guide faculty if a student is unfit to work in the clinical area as well as subsequent actions that are aimed at helping students constructively address the problem.

The Semester Begins

Before the start of each semester, the preceptor must review the course objectives in their entirety. This will enable the preceptor to plan the student's experience. Most hospitals will require proof of licensure, basic life support certification and other related certifications, and malpractice insurance as well as a physical exam, which includes documentation of immunization status prior to starting as a student. These documents should be maintained in a central place such as a nursing education office or an administrative office so they can be easily accessed.

A meeting should be set up with the preceptor, the student, and a university faculty member. During this meeting, the following items should be discussed at length and mutually agreed on: (1) a review of objectives and how they are going to be accomplished, (2) a schedule (dates and times), (3) the method of evaluation, (4) a review of personal and professional goals, and (5) future meeting schedules.

According to Shah and Polifroni,[7] the more specific the student is in identifying learning needs, the more helpful the preceptor can be. Keep in mind that the principles of adult learning should

Table 13-2

Knowles' Assumptions About Learning[9]
1. Adults have a need to know why they should learn something.
2. Adults have a need to be directed.
3. Adults have a greater volume and different quality of experience than youth.
4. Adults become ready to learn when they experience in their life situations a need to know or to be able to do something to perform more effectively.
5. Adults enter into a learning experience with a task-centered, problem-centered, or life-centered orientation to learning.
6. Adults are motivated to learn by both extrinsic and intrinsic motivators.

Table 13-4

Tips for the ED APN's First Day of Clinical Orientation
Orient to the environment
Ensure adequate parking
Obtain identification badge
Obtain library access
Orient to the other clinical areas outside the ED (e.g., trauma intensive care unit, radiology, laboratory, operating room)
Provide access to an office or locker space
Introduce to the staff
Cafeteria access

be utilized in working with the student. According to Knowles, an adult learning experience should be a process of self-directed inquiry, with the resources being the teachers, fellow students, and other materials being made available to the student, but these should never be imposed on.[8] Table 13-2 lists Knowles' set of assumptions about learning.[9]

It is common for graduate students to need strengthening in clinical reasoning or critical-thinking skills. Critical thinking can be described in many ways. Alfaro-LeFevre[10] defined it as purposeful outcome thinking that requires knowledge, skills, experience, and inquisitiveness about reasons behind actions, independent thinking, and sensitivity to emotions. The ideal critical thinker constantly reevaluates, self-corrects, and strives to improve. Many universities have developed courses to help students improve their critical-thinking skills. As a clinical faculty you can help the student develop these skills through various approaches (see Table 13-3).[11,12]

Table 13-3

Strategies for Improving Critical-Thinking Skills in the Graduate Nursing Student
■ Encourage use of a clinical journal
■ Create a trusting environment
■ Share previous experience
■ Foster self-evaluation
■ Present weekly case studies
■ Provide opportunities for group learning

The first day should also be reserved as a get-acquainted day. Some of the things that can be done on that day are listed in Table 13-4. It is important that the student be made to feel as welcome as possible. Hopefully this will decrease anxiety and make the learning experience more positive.

During this first meeting, it is important that ground rules are set. For example, this is the time to discuss which procedures the student may not perform unsupervised or the number of physical exams that must be conducted per day. It is essential to discuss as much as possible in the beginning to prevent any conflict during the clinical experience.

Method of Evaluation

Evaluation is a critical step in the student's clinical experience. According to the theories of adult learning, adults must be involved in the evaluation process from the beginning. Many preceptors meet formally with the student at the beginning of the day and again at the end of the day. At the beginning of the day, the plan should be set, and at the end of the day is when the evaluation process takes place. The preceptor should ask the student if the goals for the day were met. It may also be helpful to have students identify their strengths and weaknesses. This will help ensure that they are involved in the evaluation process.

The preceptor should be willing to share an assessment of the student as well. The criticism should be constructive, and the positive should always be emphasized. Evaluations are usually best received if specific examples are included that describe both the positive and negative. When this evaluation is conducted, it should be in private so the student does not become uncomfortable and anxious.

If the student identifies weaknesses, it is important to ask them to help determine what can be done to help them overcome this weakness. As a preceptor, you can suggest things that may be helpful. For example, if the student is having difficulty reading x-rays, you can arrange for the student to work with a radiologist for several days. When this is agreed on, it is important that the student know exactly what his or her goal is during the alternative experience.

Some universities may require weekly evaluations by the preceptor, the orientee, or both. In this case, time needs to be provided for this in your daily work routine, copies should be kept, and the original should be sent to the university faculty. If the evaluation were at the end of the semester, it would be wise for the preceptor to keep notes for future reference. These notes will help to make the final evaluation more accurate and meaningful to both the student and the preceptor. At the end of each evaluation session, recommendations and accolades should also be provided.

Some universities ask that the preceptor give the student a grade. This should be discussed in the beginning, and the guidelines for grading should be clear to the preceptor. The criteria may be slightly different from university to university. Some students will need to complete a project or write a paper that the preceptor will be responsible for grading. If this is the case, faculty from the university should be readily available for consultation when the need arises.

It is also important for the student to have the opportunity to evaluate the preceptor as well as the clinical experience. The preceptor should have access to these evaluations so that improvements in the experience can be made. This evaluation should be saved by the preceptor and included in the APN's evaluation.

Benefits

Shah and Polifroni's[7] study looked at the benefits to the graduate student, the preceptor, and the

organization from the APN mentoring through their contact with the university system and by exposure of the organization to the graduate student population. Rewards for the APN were in the form of clinical faculty appointments and library and computer facility privileges. The most positively reported rewards for the APN were personal and professional, including helping people to learn, passing the baton to a new generation, and giving back for what they had gained.

Martin and Riley[13] reported on a project in which they created research partnerships between graduate students and clinical nurses. Graduate students who received formal research education were expected to design research projects. Oftentimes these projects lacked meaning because of their hypothetical nature. When paired with clinical nurses, they found relevance for their research proposals by addressing the real problems identified by nurses in direct patient care. The clinical nurses got assistance with literature searches and study designs to examine problems. Utilizing the research partnership enabled both the graduate student and the clinical nurse to achieve their professional goals.

APNs are goal directed and are always looking for new and exciting opportunities to develop their practice. Universities can provide opportunities for lecturing and curriculum development for the APN. Often faculty is looking for experts in a specialty area. As an example, a local university solicited this author to lecture to the acute care NPs on caring for the victims of rape and domestic violence. These topics are a subspecialty of emergency nursing, and it is important that new students get the most up-to-date information about the management of these patients. As an ED APN, you can also offer your expertise to the faculty. Provide them with a list of topics on which you lecture or would be willing to lecture.

Many hospitals enjoy having nursing students because education is usually a major part of their mission as well as being helpful in recruitment. Many APN students will choose to work in an area in which they have been educated. If their experience is positive and there is opportunity for them, they may decide to take advantage of the opportunity and become employed by the hospital.

As an APN it is important to build a network of support around you and your practice. Many times university faculty will have an interest in clinical research, and an APN in a hospital setting who has little experience with research but has the desire can develop research projects and publishing opportunities that may not have been available to them without the support of the university.

Additional benefits of preceptoring an APN include additional educational offerings for the staff by the student and initiation or completion of projects for the units such as rewriting or updating policy and procedure manuals, protocols, and standards of care. The APN student may also be an asset to hospital- or unit-based committees by bringing a unique perspective. For example, when hospitals are preparing for a Joint Commission for Accreditation of Hospitals Organization survey, it is helpful to have staff on the committee who have had a recent survey or have insight into some of the evaluation criteria and standards.

Conclusion

The APN can be the most precious resource for many hospitals, patients, and families. It is important that they be mentored correctly and taught how to maintain standards of care during a very turbulent time in health care. The future of nursing and advanced practice is in the hands and minds of our new nurses, and as APNs we must take the responsibility to educate and develop them.

REFERENCES

1. Fralic, M. (1988). Nursing's precious resource: The clinical nurse specialist. *Journal of Nursing Administration, 18*(2), 5–6.
2. Lambert, V., McDonough, J. M., Ponds, E. F., & Billue, J. S. (1995). Preceptorial experience. In B. Fuzard (Ed.), *Innovative teaching strategies in nursing* (2nd ed., pp. 191–194). Gaithersburg, MD: Aspen.
3. Stewart, B. M., & Krueger, L. E. (1996). An evolutionary concept analysis of mentoring in nursing. *Journal of Professional Nursing, 12*(5), 311–321.
4. Larrabee, J. (2001). Achieving outcomes in a joint-appointment role. *Outcomes Management for Nursing Practice, 5*(2), 52–56.
5. Duffy, M. (2001). Arranging for clinical affiliations. *Journal for Nursing Staff Development, 17*(1), 41–43.
6. Spier, B. E., Matthews, J., Jack, L., Lever, J., McHaffie, E. J., & Tate, J. (2000). Impaired student performance in the clinical setting: A constructive approach. *Nurse Educator, 25*(1), 38–42.
7. Shah, H., & Polifroni, C. (1992). Preceptorship of CNS students: An exploratory study. *Clinical Nurse Specialist, 6*(1), 41–46.
8. Knowles, M. S. (1980). *The modern practice of adult education from pedagogy to andragogy.* Chicago: Follett.
9. Knowles, M. S. (1987). *Training and development handbook: A guide to human resource development.* New York: McGraw-Hill.
10. Alfaro-LeFevre, R. (1999). *Critical thinking in nursing: A practical approach.* Philadelphia: Saunders.
11. Youngblood, N., & Beitz, J. (2001). Developing critical thinking with active learning strategies. *Nurse Educator, 26*(1), 39–42.
12. O'Neill, E. S. (1999). Strengthening clinical reasoning in graduate nursing students. *Nurse Educator, 24*(2), 11–15.
13. Martin, K., & Riley, J. K. (2002). Creating a research partnership: Graduate students and clinical nurses. *Nurse Educator, 27*(1), 3–5.

14

COMPETENCY

Suzanne Rita, RN, MSN

Health care today prides itself in the competent, high quality of care that its employees provide to patients and their families. Validation of competency from initial training through annual review and continuing education is essential to maintain a high quality of care. In the emergency department (ED), this becomes an immense challenge because the nursing staff must be competent in many areas of care covering patient populations of differing ages and cultures and a constantly changing environment of high technology. An organized competency program ensures verification of the knowledge and skills necessary for validation of the competencies of the ED nurse. This chapter will discuss competency, including the establishment of competency behaviors, suggestions to facilitate demonstration of these behaviors, use of competencies to evaluate performance, and strategies to maintain ongoing competencies.

Competency

Competency is defined as the ability to perform. However, nurses refer to competency as more than performance abilities. Along with performance, the nurse must demonstrate the application of knowledge, interpersonal communication skills, decision-making abilities, and psychomotor skills as expected for the nursing practice role.[1] Del Bueno's definition of competent adds the critical-thinking component. This model creates an emphasis on critical thinking and decision making, not just on task completion.[2] Del Bueno wrote extensively about competency-based nursing orientation—a program she and her colleagues developed by which managers and/or educators establish a set of behaviors that staff are required to perform at the most basic level. Needs assessment tools were generated from these competencies to determine the education that the new

nurse would require during the orientation process. Also involved in this process was the use of several different teaching strategies. Benner, Tanner, and Chesla[3] expanded the concept of competency. Using the Dreyfus model for skill acquisition and development, they described levels of competency in which a nurse moves from the use of abstract thinking to the use of intuition to make decisions. These levels are novice through expert and are further described in Table 14-1. The understanding of the novice-to-expert concept is essential to the understanding of the concept and use of competency. Zhang et al. report that interpersonal understanding is the most important characteristic of good nursing practice.[4]

Regulatory agencies support the value of competent practitioners. The Joint Commission on Accreditation of Healthcare Organizations addresses competency in the standard entitled *Management of Human Resources/Competence Assessment*. Furthermore, a separate standard (HR.4.2) focuses on the definition and evaluation of clinical staff performance and on whether the staff is competent to perform the role they are assigned.[5] Identification of what is a competent staff member and the relationship of this assessment to their identified learning needs is the key to a competent workforce.

Developing Competencies

A nurse is competent if he or she has the appropriate knowledge, skills, and training to deliver quality, safe patient care. Competencies are developed to assess, achieve, and maintain the knowledge and skills that are appropriate to the care delivered by the team member. Competency outcomes are based on performance measures in the job description, which are further broken down into a series of activities that is then broken down into

Table 14-1		
Benner's Model of Nursing Competency		
LEVEL	EXPERIENCE	DECISION MAKING
Novice	0–6 months	■ Limited decision-making capability ■ Task oriented ■ Depends strongly on rules and policies to guide their practice ■ Can identify pieces to the care of the patient but due to lack of experience cannot synthesize the pieces into a total care model
Advanced beginner	6 months–2 years	■ Cannot anticipate the life threat of a situation ■ Lacks flexibility; cannot determine changes to plan of care if needed ■ Can begin to piece together information but continues to rely on protocol and procedures to assist with decisions ■ Has no difficulty with task accomplishment
Competent	At least 2 years	■ Able to plan for changes in patient's status and can make decision to deal with these changes ■ Can anticipate the patient's needs
Proficient	At least 2 years	■ Can synthesize pieces of information into a whole ■ Recognizes changes in patient's condition and can be flexible to change plan of care to meet these needs
Expert	Extensive experience	■ Is self-confident and possesses a high level of self-esteem ■ Focuses on information that is important; can sift out extraneous information that is not necessary to make a decision; not task oriented ■ Uses extensive experiences to make decisions about patient care ■ Rapidly anticipates the plan of care to meet the individual patient's plan of care ■ Family oriented

single observable tasks. It is expected that the nurse not only can perform the task but can also identify the purpose of the task. The nurse must also be able to understand the outcomes, both expected and unexpected, to the completion of the task. When developing competencies, performance standards are used as the basis for standard of care. Resources available to identify skills include *The ENA's Standards of Emergency Nursing, ENA's Orientation to Emergency Nursing, Emergency Nursing Core Curriculum,* and the *ANA Code of Ethics.* Also useful is the integration of nursing policy and procedures, clinical pathways, and standards of care into the competency assessment tool. Areas of core competency are listed in Table 14-2.

Once the core competencies are identified, the appropriate evaluation method must be identified. Although self-reporting is essential for identification of learning needs, this is the least successful and least accurate method for evaluation. The most effective evaluation method is observation by either the manager or the preceptor. Table 14-3 lists other measures to evaluate competency.[6]

In orientation, a competency tool should be implemented that contains all the core competencies necessary to provide safe, basic care in the ED. The preceptor is essential in the success of orientation. The preceptor must be totally engaged in the professional development of the preceptee. The preceptor must also clearly understand the goals of orientation. It is the preceptor who takes on the responsibility of validating the competency of a new employee during the process of orientation. The orientation competency

Table 14-2
Core Competencies
1. Patient plan of care 2. Age-specific knowledge and skills 3. Safe medication administration 4. Blood administration 5. Safe use of equipment 6. Safety practices 7. Safe performance of common ED procedures 8. Decision making and priority setting 9. Delegation skills 10. Skills that are low volume, high risk

Table 14-3
Competency Evaluation Methods[6]
1. Observation
2. Competency criterion tools
3. Posttest
4. Psychomotor skill demonstration/return demonstration
5. Computer-based education
6. Simulations
7. Peer review
8. Case presentations/patient care rounds
9. Self-learning packets

checklist tool should be completed during the orientation process. At the completion of the orientation period, a written evaluation of the new employee should be developed. The manager should write this plan with input from the preceptor, clinical nurse specialist (CNS), and new employee. The document should include the strengths and weaknesses of the new employee and an evaluation of the knowledge, skills, and behaviors necessary to perform the job of staff nurse. A developmental plan for the new employee should be developed to promote continuing competency and professional development.

Maintaining Competencies

Once competency has been established, it is paramount to maintain continued competency. Most educators believe that competency can be evaluated by exception. This assumption allows the manager/CNS to validate competency of frequently occurring skills during real-life situations. Therefore, only low-volume, high-risk competencies must be repeated at intervals to maintain competencies.[7] Skills that should be reviewed at least annually include the following categories.

1. Quality improvement issues/risk management issues
2. Skills that coincide with the institution's goals and initiatives
3. New skills
4. New equipment
5. High-volume, high-risk procedures
6. Low-volume, high-risk procedures

Remember, some of these skills will be universal to ED nursing. For example, a low-volume, high-risk skill could be normal delivery of a neonate. Other skills may need to be institution specific, such as review of hospital-based goals on the performance improvement activities related to ED care of the patient experiencing an acute myocardial infarction.

All of the preceding skill categories can be reviewed at an annual "Skills Day," or an ED may choose to review one or two skill categories periodically throughout the year. Techniques used to support skills competency validation include demonstration and observation, self-learning packets and videos, computer-based training, or simulations. Each skill competency must include measurable outcome objectives and valid evaluation tools.

The skills to be reviewed should be reevaluated by the manager or CNS annually to ensure that new techniques and procedures are being validated. Ultimately, validation of competency is the responsibility of the nurse manager.

REFERENCES

1. National Council of State Boards of Nursing. (1997). *Definition of competence and standards for competence.* Chicago: Author.
2. del Bueno, D. J., Griffin, L., Burke, S., & Foley, M. (1990). The clinical teacher: A critical link to competence development. *Journal for Nurses in Staff Development, 6*(3), 135–138.
3. Benner, P., Tanner, C., & Chesla, C. (1992). From beginner to expert: Gaining a differential clinical world in critical care nursing. *Advances in Nursing Science, 14*(3), 13–28.
4. Zhang, Z., Luk, W., Arthur, D., & Wong, T. (2001). Nursing competencies: Personal characteristics contributing to effective nursing performance. *Journal of Advanced Nursing, 33*(4), 467–474.
5. Joint Commission on Accreditation of Healthcare Organizations. (2002). *Management of human resources/ competence assessment.* Retrieved September 13, 2002 from http://www.jcaho.org
6. Rita, S. (1997). Competency based nursing orientation. In R. F. Salluzzo, T. A. Mayer, R. W. Strauss, & P. Kidd (Eds.), *Emergency department management: Principles and applications* (pp. 692–695). St. Louis, MO: Mosby.
7. Rusche, J. D., Besuner, P., Parusch, S. K., & Berning, P. (2001). Competency program development across a merged healthcare network. *Journal for Nurses in Staff Development, 17*(5), 234–240.

PART FIVE

RESEARCH

15

USING RESEARCH TO GUIDE PRACTICE: EVIDENCE-BASED PRACTICE

Doris A. Rasmussen, MSN, RN, CCRN, CEN, CS, CCNS

Evidence-based practice (EBP) is a term used in various disciplines to support using clear research findings to defend clinical practice that will achieve the best outcome. This has particular significance for those in a health care system focusing on patients, payers, accrediting bodies, and government agencies.[1] The concept of EBP is not new; in fact, Florence Nightingale clearly identified an evidence-based framework in 1891. Nightingale introduced the concept of EBP when she investigated causes of high mortality, analyzed data, and made recommendations for reform.[2] What has clearly affected the development and use of EBP in health care has been advancement of technology, flow of information, and consumer demand.[3] Application of these findings to practice and the ability to measure outcomes has spurred the use of EBP in health care.

EBP, as it applies to nursing, indicates the most appropriate framework to obtain the best outcomes for clinical practice and to reduce costs. However, before this term can be operationalized, it must be defined. In the literature, there is a consistent theme to the definition: EBP is the process of systematically finding and appraising research for the conscientious, explicit, and judicious use in making clinical decisions.[4,5] To use an EBP framework, clinicians have the responsibility to investigate sensitive issues associated with risks and benefits related to practice, outcomes, and costs.

Consumers and insurers of health care demand competent care supported by research findings that demonstrate effectiveness. Interventions related to the process of care must also be validated to determine appropriateness for clinical practice and contributions to patient care outcomes.

As a process, EBP is concerned with finding, appraising, and applying scientific evidence for the treatment and management of health care. To improve the effectiveness of these services, the following areas have been identified for consideration to move practice forward.

1. Create a scientific culture to emphasize scientific inquiry.
2. Organize and systematize knowledge for dissemination.
3. Utilize a formal system for change to analyze quality of care and to support practice changes.
4. Identify incentives to encourage effective clinical practice.[6]

Nurses have the opportunity to demonstrate leadership in directing clinical practice decisions that are evidence based. To achieve this, scientific knowledge should be the foundation for clinical practice to satisfy consumers, providers, and insurers of health care. This requires commitment by individual nurses for their own best-practice endeavor and to ensure credibility as a profession.[3]

Process

To maintain the highest standards of care that are cost effective requires understanding the benefits as well as the risks of advances in medical technology. Also, it is necessary to determine which patients would benefit most from available treatments. Practitioners can approach evaluation of the literature with consistency to obtain sound evidence for best practice by using the following steps.

1. Reflect on practice and areas of concern.
2. Formulate a well-balanced question.
3. Track down relevant articles for the best possible evidence.

4. Critically appraise the literature findings for validity.
5. Change practice if indicated by research.
6. Write new practice guidelines.
7. Disseminate findings.[7,8]

Reflecting on Practice

When considering practice changes, priorities are given to those populations classified as high volume, high risk, and high cost. Assessing current practice requires reviewing the effectiveness of a treatment intervention and its ability to cause something to happen. At the same time, it is important to determine if there is a positive or negative effect and what impact this has on efficiency, cost, and clinical effectiveness.

Efficiency is an aspect of health care delivery associated with structure and process variables. Usually, this is determined by the ratio of a system's output to its input. For example, you may have an efficient system, but it may not be effective as reflected by patient outcomes. State-of-the-art equipment and testing capabilities may be in place, but proper sequencing of the process of care is lacking. Also to be considered is the educational component necessary for staff to become competent regarding a new intervention or a new patient population. Costs incurred for new technology and required staff education are factors to consider when determining the effectiveness of a treatment intervention or a practice change.

Cost-benefit is a term used to compare an intervention's costs and benefits. For example, if benefits in financial terms were greater than the costs, a cost-benefit analysis would suggest that the treatment is worth doing. An analysis of cost-benefit is difficult to conduct and requires direct costs as well as less-tangible costs and benefits to the patient and society at large. This analysis is difficult, but it is considered to be essential when dealing with limited financial resources, such as state-funded health care systems. By obtaining this information, decision makers are able to make the hard choices to achieve the greatest good for the least cost to enhance clinical effectiveness.[9]

Clinical effectiveness encompasses the concepts of effectiveness, efficiency, efficacy, and benefit. From this is derived its definition:

The extent to which specific interventions, when deployed in the field for a particular patient or population, do what they are intended to do. That is, maintain or improve health and secure the greatest possible health gain from the resources available.[9]

When considering a clinical effectiveness initiative, decisions regarding clinical services and care are driven by clinical and cost effectiveness and their effect on outcomes. By evaluating on this basis, the greatest health gain can be secured for the resources available to become an integrated part of health care delivery.

Formulate a Well-Balanced Question

The relevance of clinical information depends on the frequency with which a problem is presented. If a clinician does not perceive a concern regarding a practice issue, the information relating to this issue is of minimal value. Specific steps that provide guidance to ensure the question is well thought out and well balanced include:

1. Describe the characteristics of your patient/population.
2. Define the intervention you are considering.
3. Define, if necessary, a comparison maneuver.
4. Identify the desired outcome.[7]

To assist in remembering these steps, the acronym PICO may be of use. The components of this acronym are: P-patient, I-intervention, C-comparison, and O-outcome. An example of a question inclusive of PICO is: In a patient suspected to have bacterial endocarditis on the basis of positive blood cultures, would transesophageal echocardiogram be a more sensitive test than transthoracic echocardiogram for identifying valvular vegetations and abscess? Posing a question requiring specific information will save time and resources when conducting a literature search.[7]

Literature Search for Evidence

Clinicians are faced with the challenge of filtering and synthesizing numerous articles published annually into manageable information. Frequently, the barrier in communication between clinician and researcher is the language used to present research findings. When this occurs, there is a delay in getting research into practice. Accessing literature for evidence-based nursing has become easier for clinicians because of the number and quality of sources appraised and summarized for clinicians. Also, strategies can identify research based on an appropriate design to answer a particular clinical question. Nurse researchers use a multidisciplinary approach to retrieve and integrate evidence into professional nursing practice. Advanced practice nurses (APNs) must expand and refine their skills in conducting literature searches that are pertinent and effective to contribute evidence for best practice in nursing. Several databases (Table 15-1) are available that are relevant to nursing and can provide evidence to strengthen clinical practice.[10]

Table 15-1	
Databases[10]	
CINAHL (Cumulative Index to Nursing and Allied Health Literature)	■ Includes aspects of nursing, allied health, alternative health, and community medicine ■ Indexes a number of nursing-related books and book chapters that are not indexed in other sources ■ Provides articles for several regional nursing journals and some government documents ■ Added feature: Their citations have abstracts, and many will list the references for the publication
MEDLINE	■ Majority of articles in this database include abstracts; however, there may be review articles, letters, and editorials ■ Free access through PubMed (http://www.pubmed.gov) ■ Added feature: Embedded links from the citations to electronic full-text copies of the articles
Cochrane Library	■ Resource sponsored by the Cochrane Collaboration, (http://hiru.mcmaster.ca/cochrane/); included are a number of databases that direct health care professionals to information that supports decisions for treatments and interventions ■ Cochrane Database of Systematic Reviews includes full-text systematic reviews that are listed as protocols. The full-text reviews are indexed and abstracted in both the CINAHL database and MEDLINE, with MEDLINE references having links to the Cochrane Database from the citations.
PsycINFO	■ Database of the American Psychological Association ■ Includes all areas of psychology, including many applications to other fields of study. More thoroughly indexed, and it is a good choice for reviewing qualitative research. This is of benefit when searching the mental health nursing literature for aspects of human behavior and research related to patient and family responses to clinical treatments. ■ Other advantages of this database include having access to dissertations, technical reports, books, and book chapters
Evidence-Based Nursing	■ Journal published quarterly; tool to promote awareness of advances in research as it relates to nursing practice ■ Authors are clinical experts in a given field, who summarize research articles and present the information in an extended abstract format, including commentary ■ There are only a limited number of journal articles reviewed for this publication for any one topic; however, it is recognized for its high quality
Educational Resources Information Center (ERIC)	■ Database that provides coverage of the field of education, including training and development ■ Allows for retrieving full-text ERIC digests and documents. These documents include books, book chapters, research reports, conference papers, and other presentation documents. ■ Research libraries often subscribe to the ERIC microfiche service to provide an access to a majority of the documents in this database

When conducting a literature search, it will help the searcher retrieve the highest levels of evidence for a particular clinical question if various levels of evidence are identified. Adding methodology terms and clinical filters to subject terms will result in efficient and optimal retrieval to find the highest level of evidence in answering clinical questions. Table 15-2 and Table 15-3 present levels of clinical evidence related to primary and secondary literature.

Appraise Literature for Validity

Nurses are compelled to seek literature that supports best practice and is evidence based. There is an abundance of health care information in print and online that can be readily accessed. However, this does not give merit to the data to be scientific, based on validity, reliability, and generalizability of the findings. You must always question whether the research results can be applied safely to clinical practice. This requires skill and diligence to conduct a review and critique of the literature.

Critical appraisal is made easier and more efficient by the availability of quality checklists or guidelines. The framework to critique studies addresses three fundamental areas designed to assist in providing better care to patients.

1. Are the results of the study valid? Do the results reflect the true size and direction of treatment effect? Was the study conducted to minimize bias and lead to accurate findings?[11]

It is possible that the different treatments conditions actually do produce different effects and therefore cause the individual's scores to be higher or lower in one condition than in another. Remember, the purpose of the experiment is to determine whether or not a treatment effect does exist.

Questions related to determining validity of a study are classified as either primary or secondary. Primary questions include

1. Was the assignment of patients to treatment randomized, and was the randomization concealed?
2. Was follow-up sufficiently long and complete?

Table 15-2

Levels of Clinical Evidence in the Primary Literature		
TYPE OF QUESTION	TYPE OF STUDY/METHODOLOGY	MEDLINE FILTER
Therapy	Double-blind Randomized control trial	Randomized control trial (pt), double (tw) and blind (tw), EXP clinical trials
Diagnosis	Controlled trial	Sensitivity and specificity (MH) EXP diagnosis
Prognosis	Cohort studies Case control Case series	EXP cohort studies (MH) Prognosis (MH) Survival analysis
Etiology	Cohort studies	EXP cohort studies (MH) Risk (tw)
Prevention	Randomized control trial Cohort studies	Randomized control trial (pt) Cohort studies (MH) Prevention and control (sh)
Quality improvement	Randomized control trial	Randomized control trial (pt) Practice guideline (pt) Consensus development conference (pt)

Legend: *pt-publication type; tw-text word; EXP-explode-search this term and all subordinate terms; MH-MeSH heading and subheading assigned to national indexes; sh-subject heading; AND-list of articles with term 1, list of articles with term 2, articles with both lists; OR-articles in either list*

Reprinted with permission from University of Illinois at Chicago. (n.d.). *Is all evidence created equal?* Retrieved August 13, 2002 from http://www.uic.edu/depts/lib/lhsp/resources/levels/

Table 15-3

The Secondary/Filtered/Synthesized Literature Outcome Products of Evidence-Based Medicine

FILTERED/SYNTHESIZED INFORMATION	DESCRIPTION/DEFINITION	HOW TO FIND

Systematic Reviews	■ Differ from traditional review articles in that conclusions are evidence based rather than commentary
	■ Start with a clearly articulated question
	■ Use explicit, rigorous methods to identify, critically appraise, and synthesize relevant studies
	■ Appraise relevant published and unpublished evidence before combining and analyzing data
	■ Include description of how primary data sources are identified
	■ Individual studies assessed for validity
		■ Cochrane Collaboration
		  □ Cochrane Database of Systematic Reviews
		  □ York Database of Abstracts of Reviews of Effectiveness
		  □ Cochrane Controlled Trials Register
		  □ Cochrane Review Methodology Database
		■ In MEDLINE:
		  1. Review [pt] AND medline [tw]
		  2. (Quantitative OR Systematic OR Methodologic)
		    AND (Review OR Overview)
		  3. In PubMed Clinical Queries "Systematic Review" is available as a limit option

Meta-analyses	■ Specific methodologic and statistical technique for combining quantitative data
	■ A type of systematic overview
		■ Cochrane Databases
		■ In MEDLINE:
		  1. Meta-analysis [pt]
		  2. meta-anal* [tw] OR metaanal* [tw]

Evidence-based practice guidelines	■ Gather, appraise, combine evidence systematically ■ Statements designed to assist practitioner and patient decisions ■ Developed by professional groups, government agencies, local practices ■ Structured abstract: objective, option, outcomes, evidence, values, benefits/harms/costs, recommendation, validation, sponsors	■ National Guidelines Clearinghouse—http://www.ngc.gov ■ Agency for Health Care Research and Quality—http://www.ahcpr.gov ■ MD Consult http://www.uic.edu/depts/lib/restricted/mdconsult.html

Critically appraised topics (CATs)	■ Journals that scan literature for clinically relevant studies
	■ Critically appraise the studies
	■ Provide commentary on strength of study and clinical significance
	■ One-page format
		■ EBM Reviews-ACP Journal Club (UIC access)
		■ POEMS (Patient Oriented Evidence That Matters)
		■ Locally Produced
		  □ University of Washington Pediatrics EBM CAT-Bank
		  □ University of Michigan Evidence-Based Pediatrics Critically Appraised Topics
		  □ University of Rochester Medical Center Critically Appraised Topics/Combined Internal Medicine-Pediatric Residency

Decision analyses	■ Studies that analyze decisions faced by clinicians for an individual patient, about clinical policy or a global health care policy
	■ Application of explicit, quantitative methods to analyze decisions under conditions of uncertainty
	■ Makes fully explicit all the risks and benefits of a decision
	■ Includes a decision tree
		■ In MEDLINE:
		  □ Decision Support Techniques [MH]
		  □ Cost-Benefit Analysis [MH]
		  □ Decision analysis [ti]

Legend: *pt-publication type; tw-text word; EXP-explode-search this term and all subordinate terms; MH-MeSH heading and subheading assigned to national indexes; sh-subject heading; AND- list of articles with term 1, list of articles with term 2, articles with both lists; OR-articles in either list*

Reprinted with permission from University of Illinois at Chicago. (n.d.). *Is all evidence created equal?* Retrieved August 13, 2002 from http://www.uic.edu/depts/lib/lhsp/resources/levels/

3. Were patients analyzed in the groups to which they were initially randomized?

The purpose of creating groups by randomization is for the groups to be created that are similar in all respects except for the exposure to the intervention. Through this process, known and unknown factors, such as demographics and disease severity, that could influence results are evenly distributed among groups. This information can be found in the methodology section of a study to describe how randomization was done.

For appraisal of follow-up, consideration is given to two components. The first is the length of time the patients are followed to determine the results of their treatment. This requires a certain amount of judgment of whether the duration of follow-up was sufficient related to the specific health problem. The follow-up phase should be given adequate time to detect a clinically important effect, if indeed it does exist.

The second component is for every patient initially admitted to the study to be accounted for at completion. For example, if the dropout rate differs between the intervention and control groups, this would make the study suspect. To alleviate this, a sensitivity analysis by the authors is required to identify and categorize causes of why participants did not complete the study.

Analysis of the patients should be done in the groups to which they were originally randomized. This is called "intention to treat analysis." To determine this, the reader can look for a statement that intention to treat analysis was done and can verify this by checking that the numbers presented in the analysis are close to the numbers initially randomized. Once the primary questions are answered, a more sensitive inquiry is required using the secondary questions.

Secondary questions related to validity include

1. Were patients, clinicians, outcome assessors, and data analysts unaware of (blinded to or masked from) patient allocation?
2. Were participants in each group treated equally, except for the intervention being evaluated?
3. Were the groups similar at the start of the trial?

Patients, clinicians, outcome assessors, and data analysts should be unaware of patient treatment allocation. Research studies can be labeled single, double, or triple blind, depending on how many groups of people are unaware of the treatment allocation. If patients are knowledgeable about which treatment group they are assigned to, it can contribute to heightened sensitivity to treatment effects. This can be avoided by use of a placebo that seems identical to the treatment being implemented. It is not always possible for patients, clinicians, and outcome assessors to be blinded to a treatment group; therefore, the data analysis should be done using coded data with no identification of treatment groups. Consequently, when scrutinizing studies, look for evidence that groups involved in participating and conducting the study were blinded to patient allocation. Wherever blinding was not possible, look for evidence that the researchers took steps to minimize bias.

Treatment of each group should be equal, with the only difference between the study groups being the treatment in question. It is important to not undermine this principle by implementing "cointerventions" to one group and not to the other. To prevent this, the clinicians need to be unaware of the allocation to ensure that cointerventions will not be delivered to only one group. When reviewing randomized trials, look carefully for the descriptions of the interventions received by all groups. This is of particular concern where clinicians are not blinded to allocation.

Because of the process of randomization, the groups should be sufficiently similar at the start of the trial. The baseline characteristics of the participants in each group should be described and determined to have an influence on the outcome of interest. If imbalances in baseline characteristics exist after randomization, statistical techniques can be used to adjust for these differences.[11]

2. What were the results? How large was the treatment effect? How precise was the treatment effect?[11]

To satisfy the reader regarding results of a randomized controlled trial, take into account both the size of the treatment effect and whether the treatment effect is precise. When analyzing the treatment effect, look beyond the p value because the information may be of limited usefulness if the number of participants in each group is small. The same data can be expressed in alternative ways to provide more informative data. First, consider relative risk reduction (RRR), which is the proportional reduction in rates of bad outcomes between experimental and control groups. This is calculated by the control event rate (CER) minus experimental event rate (EER) and divided by the CER ((CER minus EER)/CER). The second is absolute risk reduction (ARR), which is the CER minus EER. ARR demonstrates how much of the effect is the result of the intervention itself. The third approach is to report the number needed to treat (NNT), which is the inverse of the ARR. NNTs, when properly presented, include a description of the follow-up time and also the 95% confidence interval around the NNT estimate.

3. Will the results help me in caring for my patients? Are the patients in the study sufficiently similar to my patients? Are there risks or harms associated with the treatment that may outweigh the benefits?[11]

After reviewing the results of treatment effects, it is important to consider whether the difference is clinically important. There are occasions in which a statistically significant difference is not important because the outcome has no relevance or the difference is too small to require a practice change. Also, there are trials in which statistically significant differences are not determined. Information from these studies can be useful if they were large enough to detect a significant difference if one existed.[12]

Another aspect of reviewing research results is how precise the estimate of treatment effect is. The true effect of a treatment can never really be known; however, the results of trials are used that are estimates of effect. Confidence intervals are a statistical tool used to communicate the magnitude of the uncertainty surrounding the size of the treatment effect. A confidence interval of 95% represents the range in which it is certain that the true value lies. If the range is wide, the estimate lacks precision; conversely, if the range is narrow, the precision is high, attributing more confidence

to the results. After critiquing the study results for validity and treatment effect, the next area of concern is the relevance of the findings to improve clinical practice.

The purpose of implementing evidence-based nursing is to provide patient care based on appropriate research findings. Therefore, the clinician must be able to make some judgment of the results contributing positively to clinical practice changes for the selected population in your institution. Look at the characteristics of the patients in the study and those in your clinical practice for similarity or not to give compelling reasons for applying the results.

Another area of concern is that of feasibility in our health care system. Whether this is a primary care or tertiary care system is going to make a difference in the level of care provided and the patient volume. Also, the cost of the intervention and funds for training and equipment need to be included in the decision when making a practice change.

When reviewing randomized clinical trials, it is common for researchers to use various outcome measures for different elements of the participants' responses to treatment. These measures may include quality of life and costs as well as direct measures of the specific health care treatment or prevention. For readers of randomized clinical trials, it is important to identify the intervention and the patient or community for which it was intended. Other outcome measures of concern are reporting of adverse effects experienced by participants in the study and the cost effectiveness of interventions. These aspects can be taken into consideration by clinicians to comprehensively appraise the impact of outcomes for clinical application.[12]

Using Research to Change Practice

Practice development requires a culture in which ideas, innovations, and research are valued. This environment is also necessary to implement change or maintain practice to enhance patient care. Practice development has been defined as a participative client-centered process that integrates research and practice using a range of facilitative methods. Although this process is rooted in response to patient needs, there is also a response to the political context to bring about health policy changes.[13]

APNs are in an excellent position to champion this process because of their practice roles. They have the opportunity to provide connections for patient-focused, outcome-based care delivery within a health care system.[14] One conceptual framework for evaluating the impact of role performance in nursing practice includes the elements of structure, process, and outcomes. Therefore, it is necessary to have champions representative of these areas to have a strong collaborative foundation. Such individuals may carry a managerial responsibility, function in a clinical specialty role, or have access to fiscal and human resources.[13]

In reviewing this framework, structure includes such characteristics of the organization as physical setting, operational policies, architecture, standards, resources, equipment, and health care personnel. Process is used to describe those activities performed by the staff that either directly or indirectly affect the quality and quantity of practice. Outcome is the end result or consequence of the treatment, intervention, or service provided to make a change in the patients' care and subsequent health status.[14]

APNs have the opportunity to lead efforts to create practice environments and systems that support EBP. An example of a structure element for participation by the APN is a clinical practice committee, which may include unit-based practice councils or a component of clinical care management. The system component has the directive to develop, implement, and evaluate clinical practice guidelines, policies, procedures, standards of care, and practice to integrate EBP. Through this system, nationally authored practice guidelines, standards of care and practice, and pathways can be modified or adopted for use within the organization.[14]

The process for dissemination of these system activities is multifaceted. This includes writing symptom-management protocols, clinical pathways, and clinical guidelines. Other process measures address monitoring the impact of the implementation of practice guidelines, identification of unit practice issues, and clinical inquiry about the EBP process. Process activities for EBP support the professional role activities of the APN. These include consultation, teaching, expert role modeling, research utilization, and expert practice.[14]

Utilizing outcome activities allows APNs to review their practice for consistency with published standards, guidelines, and best-practice recommendations. Data related to outcome variables such as length of hospital stay, utilization of resources, issues of patients' perception of care, and patient access to care and services contribute to the enhancement of competent clinical practice.[14] The impact that practice that is evidence based and grounded in clinical research contributes to quality patient outcomes has been realized by many disciplines. The next challenge is to develop, disseminate, and implement clinical practice guidelines.

Guideline Development, Dissemination, and Implementation

Clinical practice guidelines are documents that have been developed systematically to assist the practitioner to make informed decisions about appropriate management of health conditions. Guidelines for clinical practice have several purposes: (1) reduce inappropriate variations in practice, (2) promote the delivery of high-quality, evidence-based health care, and (3) provide a mechanism by which health care professionals can be made accountable for clinical activities. Multidisciplinary expert panels and professional and specialty organizations contribute to the development of clinical practice guidelines. The result is a product of research utilization efforts that represents an evolution of how decisions are determined by practitioners.[14,15]

The development of clinical guidelines can be organized into four stages. The first stage requires they be based on the best available research evidence. This requires a literature search conducted to obtain evidence regarding the appropriateness and effectiveness of a variety of clinical strategies. The second stage is guideline construction based on the research evidence. This can be done in small-group work using a multidisciplinary approach. The third stage is testing the guideline by having it reviewed by professionals not involved in its development. At this time, clarity, internal consistency, and acceptability are assessed. The final stage requires reviewing the guideline after a specified period of time and determining if it needs to be modified to include new knowledge.[16] The end result is a product that is effective and will achieve its intended purpose.

For clinical guidelines to be effective, it is recommended that they contain the 11 characteristics outlined in Table 15-4.

When the guideline is ready for use, the APN should facilitate dissemination and implementation. Dissemination is the process or method used to make the guideline available to users. This can be accomplished through several strategies, such

as publishing in professional journals, sending the document to targeted individuals, and providing an educational component. An educational intervention for a specific group is more likely to have a positive outcome regarding behavior changes. This same outcome is affected by an appropriate implementation strategy.[13,16]

The purpose of a designated implementation strategy is to ensure that users adopt and apply the guidelines for their particular use. In planning a method of implementation, consideration should be given to behavior change related to structural (staff workload and financial resources) and attitudinal factors (acceptance of the guidelines and willingness to change). Implementation strategies might be targeted at both the structure and process of care. For the clinical practitioner, giving attention to specific patient prompts at the time of consultation seems to be a powerful influence on a method of implementation. For physicians, data

Table 15-4	
Characteristics of Clinical Guidelines[13,16]	
1. Validity	■ Should be apparent if the guideline is followed as evidenced by health gains and costs predicted. This demands it be rigorously developed and consistent with current scientific evidence.
2. Cost effectiveness	■ Improvement in health care should be at an acceptable level. This can be evaluated in resource use and how it corresponds to patient outcomes.
3. Reproducibility	■ Indicates that if the same evidence were used by another guideline development group, similar recommendations would be produced
4. Reliability	■ Would occur if, given the same clinical circumstances, another health professional could apply the recommendations in the same manner. Both reproducibility and reliability are more likely to occur if the guideline is developed in a systematic and rigorous manner.
5. Representation	■ Evident by participation of key disciplines and interested persons. Consideration of patient perceptions and recommendations may be included in this category.
6. Clinical applicability	■ Meaning the target population should be defined and in line with the evidence
7. Flexibility	■ Use of the guideline allows for identifying exceptions and patient preferences to be taken into account for the decision-making process
8. Clarity	■ Should be apparent by using precise definitions and user-friendly formats
9. Meticulous documentation	■ Documentation of the process of guideline development must be maintained. This includes who took part, methods used, assumptions, and identifying the recommendations based on their connections with the evidence.
10. Scheduled review process and 11. Unscheduled review process	■ Will facilitate modification of the guideline for incorporation of new knowledge

from audits and feedback had a small but potentially worthwhile effect on behavior-implementing guidelines.[13,16]

There has been minimal research on identifying the best strategies for dissemination and implementation methods. For any one process to work well, it requires thinking related to others' settings, needs, and constraints, done in a rational manner. After all, those participating are part of the same health care system, working on the same long-term goals, perhaps in different ways. To realize such a goal requires the collaboration of participants that exhibit commitment to the importance of scientific rigor and policy relevance.[17]

Conclusions

EBP occurs with integration of the best research related to patient preferences, clinician skill level, and available resources to make valid decisions for best clinical practice. The process for this to occur requires accessing, appraising, and applying scientific evidence to support practitioners in decisions that are effective to achieve desired patient outcomes and allocation of resources. Information from the evidence is incorporated into clinical guidelines to facilitate best practice and standardization of interventions.[18,19,20]

Consider EBP to be a tool to introduce, justify, and evaluate practice. Clinical guidelines can be developed when introducing another dimension of patient care or to provide rationale for making changes in an existing process.[18,19,20] The emphasis for using EBP has been to achieve best clinical practice; however, there is another aspect to consider, which is the health care system. The system can realize benefits in the areas of compliance with government agencies, fiscal management, consumer satisfaction, and professional accountability, which in turn contribute to effectiveness and improvement.

Clinical guidelines allow for determining outcomes used by providers to measure effectiveness and cost of interventions.[20] Selected variables can be identified for measurement in the areas of structure, process, and outcomes to provide end-result findings related to specific interventions and selected populations. When EBP is utilized to support clinical guidelines, the groundwork has been put in place for outcomes management.

REFERENCES

1. Youngblut, J., & Brooten, D. (2001). Evidence-based nursing practice: Why is it important? *AACN Clinical Issues, 12*(4), 468–476.
2. McDonald, L. (2001). Florence Nightingale and the early origins of evidence-based nursing. *Evidence-Based Nursing, 4*(3), 68–69.
3. Hamer, S. (1999). Evidence-based practice. In S. Hamer & G. Collinson (Eds.), *Achieving evidence-based practice: A handbook for practitioners* (pp. 3–12). New York: Harcourt Publishers Limited.
4. Rosenberg, W., & Donald, A. (1995). Evidence-based medicine: An approach to clinical problem solving. *British Medical Journal, 310*(6987), 1112–1126.
5. Beyea, S. C. (2000). Why should perioperative RNs care about evidence-based practice? *AORN Journal, 72*(1), 109–111.
6. Walshe, K., & Ham, C. (1997). *Acting on the evidence, progress in the NHS*. Birmingham: NHA Confederation & University of Birmingham Health Services Management Centre.
7. Ghosh, A. K. (2000). Enhance your practice with evidence-based medicine. [Electronic version]. *Patient Care, 4*, 32–56.
8. Cullum, N. (2000). Users' guides to the nursing literature: An introduction. *Evidence-Based Nursing, 3*, 70–71.
9. Benton, D. (2000). Clinical effectiveness. In S. Hamer & G. Collinson (Eds.), *Achieving evidence-based practice: A handbook for practitioners* (pp. 87–107). New York: Harcourt Publishers Limited.
10. Morrisey, L., & DeBourgh, G. (2001). Finding evidence: Refining literature searching skills for the advanced practice nurse. *AACN Clinical Issues, 12*(4), 560–577.
11. Cullum, N. (2000). Evaluation of studies of treatment or prevention interventions. *Evidence-Based Nursing, 3*, 100–102.
12. Cullum, N. (2001). Evaluation of studies of treatment or prevention interventions. Part 2: Applying the results of studies to our patients. *Evidence-Based Nursing, 4*, 7–8.
13. Joyce, L. (1999). Development of practice. In S. Hamer & G. Collinson (Eds.), *Achieving evidence-based practice: A handbook for practitioners* (pp. 109–127). New York: Harcourt Publishers Limited.
14. DeBourgh, G. (2001). Champions for evidence-based practice: A critical role for evidence-based practice: A critical role for advanced practice nurses. *AACN Clinical Issues, 12*(2), 491–508.
15. Beyea, S. C., & Nicoll, L. H. (1998). Developing clinical practice guidelines as an approach to evidence-based practice. *AORN Journal, 67*(5), 1037–1038.
16. Thomas, L. (1999). Clinical practice guidelines. *Evidence-Based Nursing, 2*(2), 38–39.

17. Waddell, C. (2001). So much research evidence, so little dissemination and uptake: Mixing the useful with the pleasing. *Evidence-Based Mental Health, 4*(1), 3–5.

18. Rasmussen, D., & Barnason, S. (2000). Chest pain management: Linking tertiary and rural settings. *Nursing Clinics of North America, 35*(2), 321–328.

19. Barnason, S., & Rasmussen, D. (2000). Comparison of clinical practice changes in a rapid recovery program for coronary artery bypass graft patients. *Nursing Clinics of North America, 35*(2), 395–403.

20. Goode, C., Tanaka, D., Krugman, M., O'Connor, P. A., Bailey, C., Deutchman, M., & Stolpman, N. M. (2000). Outcomes from use of an evidence-based practice guideline. *Nursing Economics, 18*(4), 202–207.

16 | OUTCOMES MANAGEMENT

Doris A. Rasmussen, MSN, RN, CCRN, CEN, CS, CCNS

Outcomes management has come to the forefront in health care because of a paradigm, driven by research, that measures outcomes or end products of care. Those in the practice professions maintain contracts with the public and must be accountable to societal demands for care that is high quality, cost efficient, and delivered in a holistic process.[1] Therefore, practitioners will need to defend their practice performance and prove their value to consumers. Outcomes measurement provides the ability to continuously compare actual findings against desired results and choose treatment options.[2] Utilization of outcomes measurement provides a method to facilitate identification of opportunities to improve practice, to make practice changes based on research, and to reduce costs through appropriate utilization of resources and technology.

Outcomes Management

Outcomes management has been defined as the enhancement of physiologic and psychosocial patient outcomes through development and implementation of exemplary health practices and services, as driven by outcomes assessment.[1,3] This is an opportune time for advanced practice nurses (APNs) to be leaders in the realm of outcomes management. There is evidence in the literature that the quality of the nursing care process affects outcomes during and after hospitalization. However, the full extent of nursing process—outcome links is relatively understudied. If this is to be addressed, APNs must begin to implement ways to measure and improve the quality of nursing care. The health care system today requires nurses to become increasingly involved in evaluating the effects of nursing care on patient outcomes and identifying nursing care processes that produce these effects.[2]

APNs are in the best position to take the lead in conducting outcome studies based on their clinical expertise, access to subjects, master's-level research education, and a need to demonstrate the effectiveness of their own care practices.[1,4] Before beginning the process of outcomes management, conditions need to be in place to facilitate data collection and variance tracking.

Structured Care Methodology Tools

Institutions are striving to streamline processes, reduce costs of health care, and establish best-practice patterns that include an interdisciplinary dimension. The tools needed to accomplish this are referred to as structured care methodologies (SCMs) and include critical pathways, algorithms, protocols, standards of care, and order sets. Table 16-1 provides a comparison of these various tools. These statements provide practitioners with advice from recognized experts based on the most current research findings. A primary aim of SCMs is to diminish practice variations and provide data on measures to improve patient outcomes.[3,5] One tool alone may not be adequate for developing standardized practice for all episodic and aggregate patient experiences, and selection will depend on which outcomes are to be addressd.[3,5]

The purpose of using an SCM is to improve physiologic, psychological, and financial outcomes over a designated period of time utilizing the most appropriate resources. The emphasis of this process is that it is done using an interdisciplinary approach and that the tools be grounded in expert knowledge and research. The finished document should reflect the elements of time line, collaboration, patient outcomes, and quality enhancement

Table 16-1

	SCM Tools
TOOL	DESCRIPTION
Guidelines	■ Usually have a broad base ■ Contain recommendations for care pertaining to a single-discipline focus with a limited domain of care ■ May be adopted from national or specialty organizations, or developed internally by using expert opinions along with an extensive review of the literature
Protocols	■ Documents providing detailed instruction on how to implement a procedure or intervention ■ Usually limited to a specific population or in conducting research to provide a standardized approach to achieving a desired outcome
Algorithms	■ Systematic procedures that follow a logical progression based on information or patient's response to a situation ■ Have a specific focus, and can guide clinicians with selections of care depending on patient response
Standards of care	■ Used to operationalize patient care processes by providing a baseline for quality care ■ Organizations develop standards by which to measure outcomes related to a specific patient problem
Critical pathways	■ Valuable tool for charting process requiring coordinated effort of several disciplines ■ They facilitate a mechanism to identify key incidents that must occur in a predictable time frame to achieve an expected outcome
Pathways	■ Delineate necessary treatment for a specified population of patients ■ Facilitate appropriate resource use ■ A standard for comparing actual with expected outcomes
Order sets	■ Medical orders that can be used separately or with one of the SCMs previously described ■ These documents are preprinted and include research-based options for the physician to provide individualized care

of care.[3,5] Remember, a scientific method is a systematic approach to problem solving and knowledge generation, and it requires use of disciplined procedures to limit errors and ensure accurate interpretation of findings.[3]

A Model for Outcomes Management

When organizing an outcomes management program, four essential principles have been identified for inclusion. They are

1. An emphasis on standards that providers can use to select appropriate interventions
2. The measurement of patient functional status and well-being, along with disease-specific clinical outcomes
3. A pooling of outcome data on a massive scale

4. The analysis and dissemination of the database to appropriate decision makers[3,6]

To build on these principles, a systematic clinical inquiry within a cohort of patients is guided by a series of four phases, which are represented in Figure 16-1.

Phase I is the selection of the patient population within your practice arena that is to be studied. At this time, descriptive data and outcomes are identified. Outcomes are categorized as either long-term or intermediate. Long-term outcomes are measured distally, or longitudinally, at specific times following an intervention. These time frames can be at designated end points, such as 3, 6, 9, or 12 months following discharge from provider management. Outcomes that may be measured using these time frames are quality of life, resource utilization, functional status, and/or satisfaction.[1,3]

FIGURE 16-1 *Outcomes Management Model*

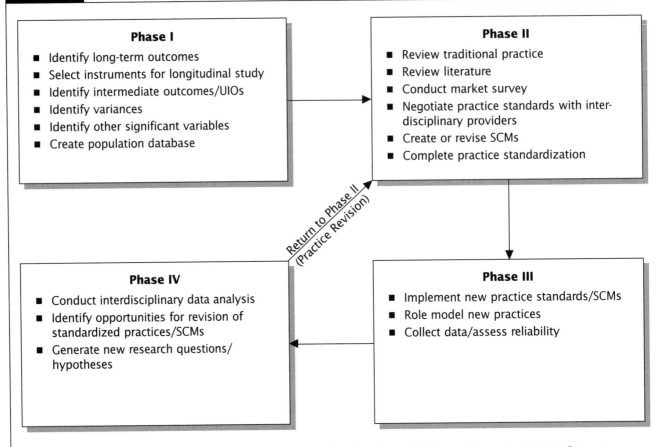

Reprinted with permission from Health Outcomes Institute, The Woodlands, TX. From Wojner, A. (2001). *Outcomes management: Applications to clinical practice* (p. 7). St. Louis, MO: Mosby.

Intermediate outcomes are measured proximally and are determined at the time of discharge from a specific level of care. The data is measured directly through documentation of outcomes attainment, untoward intermediate outcomes (UIOs) and variances. The undesired physiologic and psychosocial occurrences (UIOs) are those measured in the cohort at the completion of care. Variances refer to inefficient systems or provider practices that occur during a specific phase of care delivery.[1,3]

Once the UIOs and variances have been identified and reviewed, a determination can be made about revising them to improve processes and outcomes. Each UIO and variance should be well defined to ensure validity and reliability of the data.[1,3] Table 16-2 lists examples of UIOs and variances that may occur with the management of a patient with

asthma who presents to the emergency department (ED) in respiratory distress.

Once outcome targets have been established and definitions written, the interdisciplinary team has the task to develop an outcomes data repository. This database should support questions generated by the interdisciplinary team. The data elements identified contribute to descriptive research, which in turn supports the opportunity for improvement in clinical practice. At the completion of this process, the interdisciplinary providers have evidence to support the need for implementation of new interventions.[1,3]

Phase II consists of the development of interdisciplinary practice standards to achieve a specific outcome. There are five steps involved in this phase: (1) traditional practice patterns are analyzed, (2) literature is reviewed, (3) a market

Table 16-2	
UIOs and Variances Occurring in the Management of Asthma	
UIOs	■ Diminished gas exchange ■ Increased retained secretions ■ Decreased level of consciousness ■ Secondary pulmonary infection ■ Intubation and ventilatory support
Variances	■ Delay in door-to-drug time for nebulizer treatment ■ Provider failure to determine pre- and postpeak flow parameters ■ Provider failure to perform lung auscultation posttreatment ■ Provider failure to provide teaching or referral to community resources

survey is completed to determine alternative practice options, (4) the addition of new practices is negotiated, and (5) standardization of practice occurs.[5] SCMs are developed to address a new intervention(s) during this phase. The SCMs are derived from a combination of research, evidence-based practice, published guidelines, and expert opinion. It is important to remember that SCMs are dynamic, not static, and do not represent the final product. They are a means for performing ongoing evaluation and refining clinical practice.[1,3]

Phase III is the implementation of the new practice standards and interventions developed in Phase II. At this time, interdisciplinary provider education and credentialing are undertaken, and the new processes are piloted and implemented. In conjunction with the implementation process, provider reliability is conducted. Once this is established, data collection begins and is continued over a predetermined length of time to determine whether the intervention(s) are making a difference in the targeted patient outcome.[1,3]

Phase IV consists of analyzing data and reporting the study findings to those stakeholders and champions of this particular endeavor. During this phase, the identification of additional opportunities to improve clinical practice occurs. As a result, new research questions are generated, and the process returns to Phase II for renegotiation of practice standards and revision of SCMs.[1,3] Once the process for outcomes management is established, the next step is to identify a patient population and the outcomes associated with that population.

Patient Population/Outcomes

Early efforts related to outcomes management focused on patient populations that were high volume, high cost, and high risk. That is still true today; however, attention should also be given to selecting patients and outcomes in which a difference can be made in the care process to affect an outcome. When getting started with the outcomes management process, it is wise to select those populations with less-complex issues to measure. Experience with the process will be valuable in achieving success with populations and outcomes that are more complex.[7]

APNs are being asked to demonstrate outcomes related to their role effectiveness. Many institutions view these as cost-saving or patient-generating outcomes. Because APNs are not in revenue-generating positions, it is necessary for them to be creative to demonstrate their effectiveness and value-added benefit.[8] Opportunities for outcomes of care by the APN include symptom resolution, functional status, quality of life, knowledge of patients and families, and patient and family satisfaction. These outcomes comprise a comprehensive outcomes model: clinical, functional, costs, satisfaction, and efficiency.[4,8]

Because clinical outcomes are directly or indirectly affected by APNs, these are measures that are highly representative of the APN's effectiveness. It is important to remember that the clinical outcomes should be specifically selected. Creating a large data set is usually unnecessary and a poor use of the APN's time. To eliminate this problem, the outcomes should be clear and the variables measurable. Clinical outcomes used in nursing studies include disease-specific outcomes and will vary, depending on the patient's health problem and interventions. An essential aspect of outcomes management is to conduct the monitoring over a length of time for the effect to be properly evaluated.[4,8]

Functional outcomes include the patient's physical and emotional health, ability to participate in activities of daily living, and ability to assume their

role in the family and community. Measures of physical health status include physical functioning, role limitations, pain, general health, vitality, role limitations, social functioning, and health transition issues. The SF-36 Health Survey is an instrument frequently used to assess functional health status.[4]

When examining any outcome measure, some of the data can be translated into financial outcome. This information is of value to the organization's fiscal management department and contributes to cost and profit data. Costs can be attributed to structure such as length of stay and cost of equipment, to process such as delays in turnaround time in the ED, and to outcomes such as ineffective treatment. An outcomes study may reveal equally effective treatments but at different costs. Because APNs make decisions about treatments, there must be cost data related to the specific intervention to enhance credibility to decisions for making a change in practice.[4,8]

Satisfaction outcomes, which speak directly to the organization's customers, may include patient, family, caregivers, and physicians. Remember, satisfaction is not synonymous with quality, and consideration must be given to the customer's knowledge and the purpose of the care given. In some cases, it is difficult to determine whether the nurse practitioner (NP) or the physician has provided the care, causing the data to be somewhat unclear because of overlapping roles. Therefore, having a method to mark charts or interventions would link the care to the NP.[8] For the clinical nurse specialist (CNS), a survey could be directed to patients and those involved with a specific intervention. Questions asked would be related to process, nursing care, medical care, and outcomes of care. Physician satisfaction is another variable that is of tremendous value to both the NP and CNS. The NP has a collaborative practice agreement with the physician for providing direct patient care, whereas the CNS provides care to selected patient populations and perhaps collaborates with the same physicians. Determining outcomes related to physician satisfaction contributes to the value of APNs.

Time and efficiency are appropriate outcome measures for APNs because they can be linked with appropriate utilization of resources. For example, in the ED, tracking turnaround time of patients seen by the NP has an impact on length of stay. Also, completing patient orders and acting on the results in a timely manner contribute to efficient use of emergency services. The CNS can make use of data related to SCMs and timesaving outcomes. Tracking components of these tools as to utilization and delays of implementation and observing for errors can determine the need for improvement to structure and process issues. Time spent in a treatment room has a direct impact on the time patients spend in the waiting room, and these factors in turn contribute to patient and family satisfaction.

Building a Collaborative Practice Team

Benefits of interdisciplinary collaborative practice to patients and health care providers have been well documented in the literature. This relationship has proven to be highly positive, and both the Health Care Finance Administration and the Joint Commission on Accreditation of Healthcare Organizations have mandated collaborative planning and delivery of health services. This philosophy, however, is not valued by all health care providers.[5] A proponent for this mandate has been the need to change from payer-driven to patient-driven care to satisfy the holistic needs of patients and their families. Each patient population requires an individual with the skills required to effect change and act as a liaison to a collaborative practice team. The challenge is to select outcomes, assess the data, determine the problems for resolution, and assess the impact of change followed by renegotiating interventions.[3,7]

Participants on a collaborative practice team need to embrace the philosophy of collaboration, have a clear understanding of change theory, and support the recommendations determined by the team. The champions should be selected for each discipline based not only on their expertise, but also on their willingness to conduct business based on respect and trust to achieve positive outcomes. An ideal situation would be for all members to take off their "hats" at the table and focus on those issues contributing to best clinical prac-

tice and, ultimately, to best patient care outcomes. They need to respond to and meet the needs of health care consumers rather than impose their own personal views.

Determining Scope

Identifying the general reason for conducting an outcomes study is an initial step, but there needs to be a narrower focus on the specific aim of the study. This includes specific practices and interventions to be evaluated and the outcomes to effectively measure them. Once the outcome is identified, the specific patient variables, treatment or intervention, study design, and instruments need to be determined.

Patient variables may include demographic characteristics and patient or family resources that might influence the study and the number and type of patient comorbidities. These factors may influence patient variances and resultant outcomes.

When deciding on an intervention to be evaluated, review the literature to see if this has been tried before and in what type of setting. For example, implementing a new process of care that would shorten length (fast tracking) of stay may seem like a good thing to do. However, you first must ask if this is safe, then if it is feasible with all disciplines involved, and finally how you would evaluate it and at what specified length of time postdischarge.[9] Another area of inquiry could include evaluating whether you are practicing according to the standards of care set forth by your institution. Evaluating clinical practice and processes of care affirms that you indeed do what you say you do and provides a mechanism to detect any omissions of adhering to a patient standard of care.[10] Nursing knowledge moves forward as each researcher's experience expands on what others have done.

Data Collection Tools (Instruments)

Data collection requires a carefully thought-out plan regarding methods and selection of instruments. The instruments used will depend on the outcomes to be measured (i.e., laboratory values,

functional status, variances, patient satisfaction, or treatment protocols). Investigators may need to create their own tool if one is not already available; a review of the literature often identifies those variables that may influence the dependent variable.[6,7,11]

Whatever instrument is selected, it should be easy to use and the observations clearly presented. In addition, the validity, reliability, and responsiveness of the tool should be considered, as well as the method for data collection required by the tool and the skills and time to complete the tool.

If you are planning to benchmark your outcomes, there are sources to be aware of that can contribute to differences in outcomes:

1. Differences in the mix of patient diagnoses
2. Differences in patient severity and complexity
3. Differences in patient social and financial status
4. Differences in patient health behavior

Because of these differences, investigators have incorporated severity scores into their data collection. As a result, you are able to compare like cases and perhaps identify high-risk groups, which in turn may benefit from a higher standard of care. Severity indexing systems assign a numeric rating based on clinical information obtained from the patient's medical record and are independent of patient diagnoses.[4,6]

Data Collection Procedures

Following instrument selection, data collection procedures need to be determined. All members of the collaborative team should come to a consensus of who, where, when, and how often the data will be collected. Team members with expertise in the particular area of study should be selected to collect the data. The number of collectors should be kept to a minimum to ensure the validity and reliability of the findings. In addition, the data collectors should be given the same instruction and demonstration of the data collection procedures to ensure interrater reliability. Data should be collected at specified intervals such as daily or when a specific milestone has been achieved relative to that population. A word of caution: Do not wait until the medical record is closed and the patient is dismissed. This may

contribute to missing data entries and, therefore, loss of accuracy. Collecting the data concurrently provides a higher degree of integrity for that information.[6,7,11]

Data Entry

Data entry can be a labor-intensive responsibility depending on the number of instruments involved and pieces of data to be entered. Each variable must be formatted in a quantitative manner. Remember, all coding processes should remain consistent, including assigning missing data with a 0. A function of most statistical programs is a code within a field to designate missing data. It is a good idea to have a codebook or diary that can be maintained after creating the data fields.[6]

Consideration may be given to accessing technical assistance. Individuals assigned this role must be provided with education, including a demonstration of this process. At intervals, random checks of data entry should be conducted to ensure the data has validity and reliability.[6,7,11]

It is of great importance to have security measures in place with the understanding that all persons adhere to them. All instruments with raw data, signed consents, and all evidence of patient identification should be kept under lock and key. Consider requiring a password to access computer files and maintaining a backup system.

Data entry can be tedious and monotonous due to its repetitiveness, and there may be the tendency to get careless, which could affect the accuracy of the data. Additionally, a large complex data set may make quality control difficult to manage. To keep some semblance of control to ensure validity and reliability, the data entry process should be assessed at regular intervals. The outcome measurements are dependent on the rigor of the study design and the data entered for analysis. Therefore, if the data is not accurate and is of poor quality, clinical practice interventions cannot be validated.[6,7,11]

Analysis of the Data

Most APNs have been introduced to statistics and the research process and have conducted a data-based project. However, this may not have provided them with the expertise needed for analysis of the data and interpretation of the results. Relationships they have formed with faculty and doctorally prepared clinicians may provide access to consultants for study design and analysis issues. The availability of a statistician is extremely valuable for running statistical programs and for interpretation of the results. Many health care institutions have data managers and statisticians on staff that are available for assistance with statistics. It is important to consult with the person who agrees to assist with data analysis during the planning phase to ensure that the level of data collected and statistics used are appropriate to support a meaningful analysis.

Not all findings are going to have positive implications because some variables demonstrate a negative or nonsignificant relationship with the dependent variable. That knowledge is important for clinical practice if we are to support appropriate interventions or eliminate those that are ineffective.

Dissemination of Study Results

Any research study is meaningless unless the results are disseminated. The measurement and reporting of outcome results are of value only if this information is shared with others. Those participating on the collaborative practice team certainly need to be made aware of the study results and the process of how they were derived. The reporting should not stop there because personnel on the patient care units, physician groups, and ancillary department staff that may be affected by these findings should also be informed of them.

Content for reports can vary, depending on the purpose and the categories of data to be presented. Consider including the following areas when developing the report: (1) target audience, (2) ability to visually and narratively describe points of emphasis as they pertain to performance improvement, (3) regulatory and accreditation requirements, (4) mechanisms for benchmarking over time, (5) potential use for marketing health services, and (6) the ability to stimulate future market potential.[3]

Outcomes Measurement for the APN

Optimizing clinical practice is the overriding priority for APNs and is achieved by demonstration of competencies essential for advanced nursing practice. APN competencies include clinical expertise, critical thinking or analysis, clinical judgment or decision making, leadership and management communication, problem solving, collaboration, education, research, and program development.[12] Because EDs provide the first and often the last door between the community and the health care facility, APNs practicing in the ED need to pay close attention to competency outcome and measurement.

Outcome measures used in advanced practice effectiveness research have been categorized as care-related, patient-related, or performance-related outcomes. Care-related outcomes are those that result from the APN's involvement in direct patient care or an APN intervention. Studies have reported that the impact of care provided by APNs has ranged from lab indices to physiological and clinical symptoms. These studies have concluded that APNs perform both expanded nursing practice activities and collaborative physician-related activities. Some parameters reported include decreased length of stay, annual costs savings, time savings for staff, and decreased clinic waiting times.[13]

Patient-related outcomes of care are those outcomes that affect patient perceptions, preferences, or knowledge. Studies in this category report findings that measure the effect of the APN on patient satisfaction, patient complaints, patient knowledge, symptom management, social function, quality of life, and psychological function. The conclusions of studies in this category find APN involvement increases patient compliance with recommended treatment, decreases health care charges, decreases length of hospital stay, decreases readmission rates, and increases patient education.[13]

Performance-related outcomes include those that reflect the quality of care provided by the APN. These outcomes include quality of care, interpersonal skills, technical quality, completeness of documentation, and time spent in the role. Findings associated with performance-related outcomes include comparable care to that from physicians in the area of primary care, 98% to 99% appropriate use of prescription drugs as consistent with protocol, increased satisfaction of care reported by patients, and evidence of decreased costs.[13]

In summary, clinical and cost outcomes are improved by identifying patients at risk, closely monitoring for complications, and having a consistent APN to guide and manage the care of specified group of patients.[14] Information such as this is not only valuable as it relates to patients, it is also a means of providing information to purchasers and consumers of the quality of health care delivery at a particular institution.[15]

REFERENCES

1. Wojner, A. (1999). Outcomes management and ACNP. In P. Logan (Ed.), *Principles of practice for the acute care nurse practitioner* (pp. 99–116). Stamford, CT: Appleton & Lange.
2. Lee, J. L., Chang, B., Pearson, M. L., Khan, K. L., & Rubenstein, L. V. (1999). Does what nurses do affect clinical outcomes for hospitalized patients? A review of the literature. *Health Services Research Journal, 34*(5 Pt.1), 1011–1032.
3. Wojner, A. (2001). An introduction to outcomes management. In A. Wojner (Ed.), *Outcomes management applications to clinical practice* (pp. 3–12). St. Louis, MO: Mosby.
4. Oermann, M. H., & Floyd, J. A. (2002). Outcomes research: An essential component of the advanced practice nurse role. *Clinical Nurse Specialist, 16*(3), 140–144.
5. Cole, L., & Houston, S. (1999). Structured care methodologies: Evolution and use in patient care delivery. *Outcomes Management for Nursing Practice, 3*(2), 53–60.
6. Ellwood, P. M. (1988). Shattuck lecture-outcomes management: A technology of patient experience. *New England Journal of Medicine, 318*(23), 1549–1556.
7. Houston, S. (1996). Getting started in outcomes research. *AACN Clinical Issues, 7*(1), 146–152.
8. Burns, S. (2001). Selecting advanced practice nurse outcome measures. In R. Kleinpell (Ed.), *Outcome assessment in advanced practice nursing* (pp. 73–89). New York: Springer.
9. Barnason, S., & Rasmussen, D. (2002). Patient outcomes beyond hospitalization: Carotid endarterectomy surgical patient outcomes after a rapid recovery program. *Clinical Nurse Specialist, 16*(2), 100–105.

10. Rasmussen, D., Barnason, S., Smith, J., Epp, M., Hag, M., Gable, C., et al. (2001). Patient outcomes after peripheral revascularization surgery. *Journal of Vascular Nursing, 19*(4), 108–114.

11. Galvan, T. J. (1999). Identifying outcomes. *Nurse Practitioner Forum, 10*(4), 185–190.

12. Davies, B., & Hughes, A. M. (2002). Clarification of advanced nursing practice: Characteristics and competencies. 1995. *Clinical Nurse Specialist, 16*(3), 147–152.

13. Kleinpell, R. (2001). Measuring outcomes in advanced practice nursing. In R. Kleinpell (Ed.), *Outcome assessment in advanced practice nursing* (pp. 1–50). New York: Springer.

14. Russell, D., VorderBruegge, M., & Burns, S. M. (2002). Effect of an outcomes-managed approach to care of neuroscience patients by acute care nurse practitioners. *American Journal of Critical Care, 11*(4), 353–362.

15. Oermann, M. H., & Huber, D. (1999). Patient outcomes. A measure of nursing's value. *American Journal of Nursing, 99*(9), 40–47.

17

INTERPRETING RESEARCH

Susan A. Barnason, PhD, RN, CEN, CCRN, APRN, BC

Advanced practice nurses (APNs) are voracious consumers of research. Whether in clinical practice or academic settings, APNs strive to continuously stay on the cusp of the latest research and evidence-based practices (EBP) to optimize patient care management and to achieve improved clinical practice outcomes. The key to deriving meaningful interpretation from research is dependent on the APN's ability to interpret research findings. The impetus of this chapter is to provide APNs with a focused examination of key elements for research interpretation.

Comparison of Qualitative and Quantitative Study Designs and Data Analysis

The essence of qualitative studies is the examination and analysis of words or themes, rather than the traditional number crunching associated with quantitative study designs. All qualitative analyses use content analysis.[1] The selected qualitative research design will determine the type of data analysis. Table 17-1 provides brief summaries of some commonly used qualitative research designs and the associated data analyses usually used.[1-6]

Table 17-1	
Commonly Used Qualitative Research Designs	
Phenomenological design	Data collected are based on an individual's communication of an experience or series of experiences. The goal of the researcher is to translate the individual's communication of these experiences into an understanding and meaning of the experiences. The data analysis using this design can be either eidetic (descriptive) or hermeneutic (interpretive). Qualitative researchers using hermeneutics try to interpret the meaning of the lived human experience through both the individual's experiences and in relation to sociohistorical influences.
Grounded theory design	The goal of this study design is to generate theory through the process of concurrently collecting and analyzing data. This simultaneous process of data analysis is also known as "constant comparative" method. As data collection proceeds, data are categorized. As additional data are collected, new categories may emerge and thus are added to the list of data coding categories. The goal of this type of study is to develop theory that is grounded in the data.
Ethnographic design	The primary data are collected through subject observation and interview of key informants with the purpose of describing the culture or subculture (behaviors and value patterns) of a targeted population. The researcher analyzes the data collected from social situations or activities and categorizes those deemed to be significant into domains (symbolic categories) of the targeted culture. Researchers analyze the data from either an etic (interpretation from an outsider's view) or emic (interpretation from an insider's view) perspective. The goal of ethnographic studies is to develop cultural theories.

(continued)

Table 17-1	
Commonly Used Qualitative Research Designs (continued)	
Historical design	Historical research is used to critically appraise past events to determine how these events affect the present and future. Researchers gather data from a variety of sources (e.g., published materials, oral histories, government documents) to derive a perspective of the lives and times in the historical era of interest. Again, the data are categorized and conclusions deduced by the researcher.
Case study design	The focus of this design, using a comprehensive examination process, is to derive meaning from both commonalities and distinctive features of the targeted populations (individuals, groups of people) or an organization. Some data sources include observations, interviews, and document review. Data analysis involves linking the multiple sources of data and identifying patterns or "themes" in the data.
Focus group design	Using group interviews, this study design is intended to seek the opinions and feelings of individuals as they dialogue about a targeted issue or concern. Multiple focus groups can be used on the same topic. The group interview is led by a moderator, often a researcher, with abilities to solicit input from all group members on the topic(s) of interest. Data is analyzed by identifying response patterns and themes of the group. This qualitative technique is often used in nursing research to develop questionnaires, explore concepts, interpret discrepancies or contradictions from previous research findings, or validate previous research findings.

Designs used in quantitative research can be broadly categorized as either nonexperimental or experimental. Nonexperimental studies, which includes both descriptive and correlational studies, are used to explore patient groups or situations for purposes of characterizing the phenomena of interest, developing theory, identifying problems, or justifying current practices.[7] The studies do not involve any manipulation of variables and can reflect one point in time, explorations over time, or at multiple time points.[8] Commonly used nonexperimental designs are shown in Figure 17-1.

The other quantitative study design category is experimental, which includes both quasi-experimental and experimental studies. Experimental studies seek to control as many variables as possible to examine causality. The researcher, using experimental types of designs, actively seeks to manipulate a variable (independent variable) to determine if there is an effect on the desired outcomes (dependent variables). Commonly used quasi-experimental and experimental research designs are outlined in Figure 17-2.

Statistical analyses are used in quantitative studies to summarize study findings. Both descriptive and inferential statistics are used. Descriptive statistics depict the characteristics of the population of focus in the research study. Reporting of the data facts includes measures of central tendency, dispersion, and position within the sample or population (Table 17-2).

To determine if there are differences found in the research study, inferential statistics are used for

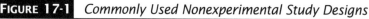

FIGURE 17-1 *Commonly Used Nonexperimental Study Designs*

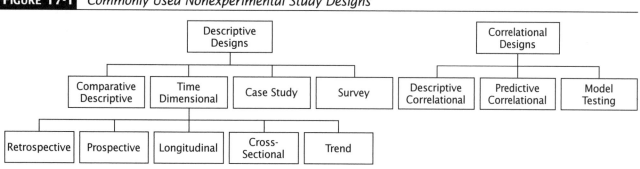

FIGURE 17-2 *Commonly Used Experimental Study Designs*

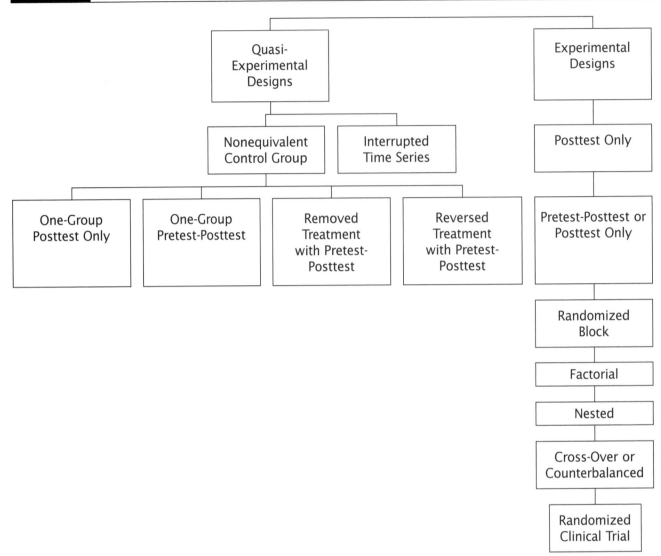

data analysis.[10] Primarily, inferential statistics are conducted to test hypotheses. All testing of hypotheses is a process of rejecting the null hypothesis. In other words, finding a statistical difference in results indicates that the null hypothesis is rejected, or the statistical difference indicates it is unlikely that the significant difference is due to chance alone. One never proves that the hypothesis is correct, but only rejects the null hypothesis.

There are two types of inferential statistics—nonparametric and parametric. Parametric statistics are the most commonly used type of statistic, which involves estimating or testing the value(s) of a parameter or measure. To use parametric statistics, users should evaluate whether the data being measured meets the criteria or assumptions to use parametric statistics. Assumptions include (1) dependent variables must be measured on an interval or ratio scale, (2) variables must be normally distributed (e.g., bell-shaped curve), and (3) variances of the variables must be homogeneous. When researchers are unable to meet all of

Table 17-2		
Descriptive Statistics		
Measures of central tendency[1,2,9]	Mean	■ Arithmetic average of a measure's finding
	Median	■ The number that divides the sample in half, or the "middle" score
	Mode	■ Most frequently occurring score or result
Measures of dispersion	Range	■ Difference between the high and low score in the sample
	Percentile rank	■ Position of a score below which a percentage of the scores occurs. The median of the scores is the 50th percentile.
	Standard deviation	■ Spread of scores around the mean; the standard deviation reflects how widely distributed the scores are for the sample
	Standard scores	■ Indicate the distance a given score is from the mean

the assumptions needed to use parametric statistics, nonparametric statistics may be used. Nonparametric statistics make less-stringent demands of the data. Especially in clinical research, it is often difficult to obtain large samples and samples that are normally distributed. Another driving force to use nonparametric statistics is related to the limitations of some of the measurement instruments used in clinical research; the measures, or tools, do not have an interval or ratio level of data, thus limiting the use of parametric statistics for the type of data generated. As a general rule of thumb, nominal and ordinal levels of data are usually evaluated with nonparametric statistics. Interval and ratio levels of measurement are evaluated using parametric statistics. Other aspects to consider when determining the use of parametric versus nonparametric statistics include how large the sample is, whether probability sampling (randomization) is used, and whether the study sample is normally distributed. Generally, when the sample is small and normal distribution of the sample cannot be inferred, it is recommended that nonparametric statistical analysis be used. Briefly, some of the more common parametric and nonparametric statistical tests are described in Table 17-3.

Nontraditional Designs and Analyses

On occasion, researchers may utilize other strategies to examine research questions or hypotheses. Other commonly used nontraditional study designs and analyses include the following:[2,8]

■ Secondary analysis: Is not a research design, but a reexamination and analysis of data collected in another study. New research questions are examined in this analysis.

■ Meta-analysis: Is not a research design, but a method of research that examines the results of numerous studies on a given topic. Statistical analyses are used to derive "overall" findings and synthesize identified research questions or problems.

■ Methodological design: A type of study design that seeks to further document the validity of measurement instruments.

■ Evaluation research design: Includes use of both quasi-experimental and experimental research designs to evaluate a clinical practice, treatment, policy, or program. May include either formative (assessment while a program or clinical practice is being implemented) or summative (assessment at completion of program or clinical practice) evaluation.

These examples of qualitative, quantitative, and nontraditional research designs assist the APN in framing the types of research designs that can be used in research studies. Research design evaluation is pivotal in determining if the research questions proposed can be appropriately addressed and therefore whether research findings from a study can be translated into research utilization or EBP.

Key Elements in Research Interpretation

The usefulness of the findings from research is dependent on the careful examination of the re-

Table 17-3		
Statistical Tests		
Parametric statistics[2,4]	*t* tests	■ Used to determine whether two group means are different when interval or ratio levels of measure are used
	Analysis of variance	■ Used to determine the difference between more than two means of a measure; again, the level of measurement is either interval or ratio
	Analysis of covariance	■ Allows the researcher to account for variables that may "confound" the findings; analysis of covariance can be used to determine the differences between two or more means of a measure
	Pearson product-moment correlation	■ Can be used to test the hypothesis regarding the relationships between data sets and between populations
Nonparametric statistics[2,9]	Chi-square	■ Can be used for nominal or higher levels of measurement and on one or more samples; the analysis determines whether the frequencies of scores fall within the range of expected frequencies within the categories
	Mann-Whitney *U* test	■ Is used to determine whether two groups differ on two sets of ranked data
	Spearman rho correlation	■ Used to determine the relationship between two variables
	Kruskal-Wallis one-way analysis of variance	■ A one-way analysis of variance for ordinal level data, which is examined by examining the rank order of data

search study. Exploring the data analysis to derive meaning from the data is the basis for research interpretation. The essential steps in research interpretation include a critique of how the data analysis is related to the following aspects: (1) research plan, (2) measurements used, (3) data collection methods, and (4) conclusions and implications of research findings.

A solid research study demonstrates clear linkages between the purpose of the study and the research questions or stated hypotheses for the study. The significance of the proposed research identifies the research problem or research statement[11] supported by other research literature. Data collection measures have a very direct relationship to the study's purpose. Measures should not only be reliable and valid, but also be relevant to both the study's purpose and research questions or hypotheses.

Both the design of the research study and the level of measurement used to collect study data drive data analyses implemented in a research study. Table 17-4 provides an overview of levels of measurement.[2,7]

Table 17-4
Levels of Measurement Used in Data Collection
Nominal Level of Measurement: Used to categorize subjects, events, or objects. Data that has mutually exclusive categories. The categories are absolute. The only type of descriptive statistic appropriate for this level of measurement is "mode."   EXAMPLES: Gender (males & females are the category of data), Marital status
Ordinal Level of Measurement: Used to demonstrate ranking of objects or events. The intervals between the categories of data may not be equal, and there is no "absolute" zero point on the scale of measurement.   EXAMPLE: Use of a Likert scale to measure satisfaction ranging from very satisfied to very dissatisfied
Interval Level of Measurement: The data intervals on a scale are equal, but there is no "absolute" zero point, but rather an arbitrary zero on the scale of measurement.   EXAMPLE: The measurement of temperature using a thermometer
Ratio Level of Measurement: The scale has equal intervals and an absolute zero value because all subjects start at zero.   EXAMPLE: The measurement of weight using a scale

Table 17-5

| Checklist to Evaluate Data Analyses Used in Quantitative and Qualitative Studies ||
QUANTITATIVE DATA ANALYSIS	QUALITATIVE DATA ANALYSIS
■ Congruency exists between data analyzed and *purpose* of the study. ■ Statistical analyses are appropriate to the design of the study and level of data measurement. ■ Data analysis findings are clearly stated. ■ Data findings are reported for each research question or hypothesis in the study.	■ Coding of data is described. ■ Strategy for data analysis is logically presented. ■ Data analysis is appropriate for *purpose* of the study. ■ Themes identified (if using narrative data) capture the essence and substance of the narrative data. ■ Analysis and conclusions derived by researcher could be interpreted similarly by another researcher (known as "auditability"). ■ Researcher has subjects review the researcher's interpretation to determine accuracy of the subjects' experiences (known as credibility). ■ Analysis is described with enough specificity to allow other researchers or clinicians to evaluate for their own practice (known as fittingness).

The researcher then interprets outcomes from data analysis. The key aspects to be considered by APNs in evaluating data analyses of the research study are summarized in Table 17-5. As an exemplar of how evaluation of data analysis was applied to a quantitative research study,[12] refer to Table 17-6.

Quantitative studies using either quasi-experimental or experimental designs use decision theory[7] to determine if results are significant. Statistically significant results either support the original proposed hypothesis or show that the findings are not likely to be due to chance occurrence alone.[1,7] Nonsignificant results may indicate that the independent variable in the study did not make a difference in the dependent variables studied. Based on the study, although there may or may not be statistically significant findings, APNs need to determine if the finding are clinically significant. For example, study findings may indicate that there were no statistically significant differences in the depression scores of two groups of patients—one group who received a treatment intervention for depression and the other being a control group. However, the improvement in the score demonstrated by the treatment group, based on other studies, was an improvement on the standardized depression instrument. Thus the clinician concludes there was some clinical significance of the findings.

The researcher deduces conclusions from data analysis summarization, which identifies knowledge gained and, in some cases, generalizations of the study. Conclusions subsequently lead to deriving implications or recognizing how study findings could be used to implement potential changes by others. Implications may also indicate that replication of the study or changes in research methods (e.g., sample, setting) may be needed before proposing changes.

Interpreting Research: Implications for APNs

Bringing about change in clinical practice requires a multifaceted effort. Infusion of new practices and the latest techniques for the management of both individual patients and aggregate patient populations is the targeted outcome. APNs are compelled to keep their practices current through ongoing review of the current literature and other sources of clinical practice standards and guidelines. To integrate EBPs into one's clinical setting, the foundation for evaluating and deriving implications of these sources is based on appropriate interpretation of research.

Table 17-6

Exemplar of Using Criteria for Data Analysis of a Quantitative Study

DATA ANALYSIS EVALUATION CRITERIA FOR QUANTITATIVE STUDIES	EXEMPLAR: EVALUATING DATA ANALYSIS OF A QUANTITATIVE STUDY[12]
1. Congruency between data analyzed and *purpose* of the study.	1. Purpose of study: "To determine most effective nursing intervention to decrease **pain** for patients with minor musculoskeletal trauma and moderate pain at triage and to examine **patient satisfaction**" (p. 124). In this study, researchers analyzed **pain ratings** and **patient satisfaction** of patients randomized to the groups (standard care, Ibuprofen, and music groups). Therefore, there was congruency between data analyzed and study purpose.
2. Statistical analyses are appropriate to the design of the study and level of data measurement.	2. This quasi-experimental study design used a numeric rating scale and verbal descriptor scale to measure pain and a Likert scale to measure patient satisfaction. Interval pain measures were appropriately analyzed using analysis of variance (ANOVA) statistical analysis to determine if there were differences in pain intensity ratings at 30 and 60 minutes after intervention, compared to baseline measures in triage. Descriptive statistics were appropriately used to report satisfaction findings in this group. Further analysis compared dichotomized patients with higher versus lower pain ratings and compared patients' perceptions of satisfaction. Statistical analysis using ANOVA was appropriately used and demonstrated that patients with "higher" pain ratings were statistically less satisfied with pain management.
3. Data analysis findings are clearly stated.	3. The analysis findings were presented using tables, figures, and narrative to augment study findings very clearly.
4. Data findings reported for each research question or hypothesis in the study.	4. Data findings were reported based on the two primary focuses of the study: pain relief and patient satisfaction with pain management interventions.

REFERENCES

1. Nieswiadomy, R. M. (2002). *Foundations of nursing research* (4th ed.). Upper Saddle River, NJ: Prentice Hall.
2. Dempsey, P. A., & Dempsey, A. D. (2000). *Using nursing research: Process, critical evaluation, and utilization* (5th ed.). Philadelphia: Lippincott Williams & Wilkins.
3. Liehr, P. R., & Marcus, M. T. (2002). Qualitative approaches in research. In G. LoBiondo-Wood & J. Haber (Eds.), *Nursing research: Methods, critical appraisal, and utilization* (5th ed., pp. 139–164). St. Louis, MO: Mosby.
4. Sullivan-Bolyai, S., & Grey, M. (2002). Experimental and quasiexperimental designs. In G. LoBiondo-Wood & J. Haber (Eds.), *Nursing research: Methods, critical appraisal, and utilization* (5th ed., pp. 203–219). St. Louis, MO: Mosby.
5. Speziale, H. J. (2002). Evaluating qualitative research. In G. LoBiondo-Wood & J. Haber (Eds.), *Nursing research: Methods, critical appraisal, and utilization* (5th ed., pp. 165–182). St. Louis, MO: Mosby.
6. Gulanick, M., & Keough, V. (1997). Focus groups: An exciting approach to clinical nursing research. *Progress in Cardiovascular Nursing, 12*(2), 24–29.
7. Burns, N., & Grove, S. K. (2001). *The practice of nursing research: Conduct, critique & utilization* (4th ed.). Philadelphia: Saunders.
8. LoBiondo-Wood, G., & Haber, J. (2002). Nonexperimental designs. In G. LoBiondo-Wood & J. Haber (Eds.), *Nursing research: Methods, critical appraisal, and utilization* (5th ed., pp. 221–237). St. Louis, MO: Mosby.
9. Bello, A. (2002). Descriptive data analysis. In G. LoBiondo-Wood & J. Haber (Eds.), *Nursing research: Methods, critical appraisal, and utilization* (5th ed., pp. 331–346). St. Louis, MO: Mosby.
10. Sullivan-Bolyai, S., & Grey, M. (2002). Inferential data analysis. In G. LoBiondo-Wood & J. Haber (Eds.), *Nursing research: Methods, critical appraisal, and utilization* (5th ed., pp. 347–363). St. Louis, MO: Mosby.
11. Haber, J. (2002). Research problems and hypotheses. In G. LoBiondo-Wood & J. Haber (Eds.), *Nursing research: Methods, critical appraisal, and utilization* (5th ed., pp. 51–75). St. Louis, MO: Mosby.
12. Tanabe, P., Thomas, R., Paice, J., Spiller, M., & Marcantonio, R. (2001). The effect of standard care, Ibuprofen and music on pain relief and patient satisfaction in adults with musculoskeletal trauma. *Journal of Emergency Nursing, 27,*(2) 124–131.

18 WRITING A RESEARCH PROPOSAL: NUTS AND BOLTS

Vicki A. Keough, RN-CS, PhD, ACNP, CCRN

Writing a research proposal sounds like an ominous task; however, approaching the proposal with a set of standards and expectations gives structure to the project, and believe it or not, writing a research proposal can even be fun. It is like putting together pieces of a puzzle. Each piece is essential to the completion of the project; however, it must be built one piece at a time. Whether or not one intends to actually conduct a major research project, request support for a clinical project, or simply conduct a small inquiry regarding data collection over a short period of time, it is necessary to prepare a written proposal.[1-13] This chapter will present general guidelines for writing a research proposal that will help give substance and structure to the research proposal.

There are three basic purposes for writing a research proposal. First and foremost, a research proposal is usually written to sell an idea for a project to a funding agency. Another purpose for writing the research proposal is to clearly describe the research plan or project, and finally, the accepted proposal will serve as a legal document between the project investigators and the funding agency.[1]

There are three basic requirements of the research proposal: (1) it must be clearly written, (2) it must be succinct and precise, and (3) most importantly, it must be persuasive.[2] Failure to meet any of these criteria usually results in rejection. The bottom line is that the funding agency needs to be convinced that the study has merit and deserves to be funded and that the research team has the ability to carry out the study.[2,3] The agency has to first and foremost want to fund the study.

Although the proposal is the first step in the implementation of the research project, a thorough understanding of the research project is necessary to complete the proposal. The research proposal starts with the initial "great idea" for a study. The idea then takes form by ruminating in the mind of the principle investigator (PI) without much form or substance. The next step is to begin writing the research proposal, which will give structure and clarity to the "great idea." The proposal gives organization and substance to a group of somewhat disconnected thoughts about how the research or project will be conducted.[1]

A research proposal should be written to stimulate interest from the funding agency. Every organization has guidelines that are specific to their needs, and these specific requirements must be addressed in the proposal.[3] The PI must have a thorough understanding of the goals of the agency that has been targeted for funding.

Know the Funding Agency

Because the ultimate goal of any research proposal is to obtain funding, it is of utmost importance that there be a good fit between the goals of the funding agency targeted and the purpose of the research project. It is up to the PI to be very familiar with the funding agency and to understand the mission and goals of the agency.[1,4] The PI should be familiar with projects that have previously been funded by the targeted agency and investigate the publications generated from such projects. Often, the name of the reviewers for each section will be available to the PI. The PI should take the time to become familiar with the publications of the reviewers and know their preferences and biases.[1,4,5] It is also recommended that the PI contact the agency staff to discuss ideas and to make sure there is sufficient interest from the agency staff before the entire project is structured.[1,4,5,6]

All grant-funding agencies publish a set of requirements or guidelines that will direct the proposal. Becoming familiar with the guidelines will give the PI further indications of whether or not there is a good fit between the targeted agency and the research project. These very important guidelines will become the blueprint for the research proposal.[1,5,6,7] Omission or weakness in any section of the guidelines will usually result in rejection of the proposal. Typically proposal guidelines include such details as abstract submissions, overview of the proposal components that will be required to apply for funding, eligibility requirements, and deadlines.[3,6,7,8,9] A general recommendation is to "read the rules, read them again, and then stick to the rules as written."[5] If the PI has any questions or concerns about the guidelines, these concerns should be dealt with immediately before progressing with proposal writing.

Another practical suggestion is to make two copies of the grant guidelines. Use one as a master copy and one as a working copy. The master copy should be filed in a safe place for reference or to clarify a section.[9]

Create a Time Line

It is common for new researchers or project directors to underestimate the amount of time that it will take to write a proposal and to end up rushing through the final stages to meet deadlines. Once the guidelines are obtained, the PI should examine the proposal carefully and determine how long each section will take to write and how long it will take to obtain supporting documents.[9] Consider planning a realistic schedule in light of current commitments, deadlines, and support. One must try to be realistic and overbudget time to allow for unexpected professional and personal issues that will also require your attention.[6,9,10]

Build a Research Team

The importance of building a strong research team cannot be underestimated. The PI should carefully consider the contributions of each member of the research team and must be sure that each team member brings an individual set of competencies and expertise to the project.[7]

If this is the first proposal for the PI, a mentor can be an invaluable resource. The mentor must have experience with grant writing. The mentor can be a valuable asset to the research team as long as there is a good fit between the mentor's research and the project being proposed.[11]

Computer Software

Become familiar with available computer software that may be helpful in grant writing, such as GrantSlam 4.0 and the Grant Application Process Planning Tool.[10,12]

Essential Elements of the Research Proposal

Not all proposals will require that the same elements be included in the body of the proposal; however, there are general sections that are standard. The essential elements of the research proposal presented in this chapter include the abstract, title, specific aims of the project (statement of the problem), significance of the study (or project), preliminary studies by the investigator, methods, protection of human subjects, literature cited, consultants, and appendices.[1-13] Appendices A through G present these various elements of a sample proposal.

Abstract

Although the abstract is really the first page of the proposal, in actuality it is the last section written. The abstract is a brief review (usually 150 to 250 words) of the proposal.[11] The abstract should include an identification of the problem and objectives and an overview of methods, cost, and amount requested by the proposal. The PI must keep in mind that this may be the only portion of the proposal that gets read if the abstract does not pique the benefactor's interest.[1]

Title

The title should reflect a brief description of the proposed study. Some things to consider in the title are the nature and subject of the research and the type of subjects with which the research is concerned (i.e., trauma patients, patients with breast cancer)[11] (see Appendix A).

Specific Aims

A summary of the research problem and basic objectives of the research are outlined in the Specific Aims section. The problem should be addressed in a clear and concise manner so that the importance of the project is understandable to the reviewer. Use data on incidence, prevalence, and sequelae of the problem to make the case for reviewers. Convince the reviewer that the project proposed is the most important research to be done.[4,5] Estimate the size of the problem and the consequences that this problem presents to Americans.[11] The writer should be careful not to make the project too large or complex, which would allow reviewers to question the manageability of the project[1,4,7] (see Appendix B).

Significance/Background

The significance or background of the research project includes a brief but thorough review of the current state of the science regarding the topic, focusing on key studies that are relevant to the proposed project. The PI should demonstrate the significance of the proposal and a strong need for the new project. The proposal needs to specify how the information discovered through the research project will contribute to nursing knowledge or nursing practice.[1,3,7] The review should include a discussion on why the proposed study is a logical step forward based on previous research. This is an opportunity to explain the theoretical and practical implications of the study and to demonstrate the knowledge of the authors.[9,11] The author should indicate how the findings from the research project will enhance nursing theory, nursing knowledge, or nursing practice.[4] Generally this section should not exceed three pages.[7] The significance section should end with the importance of your proposed study and the research questions (see Appendix C).

Preliminary Studies by PI or Investigative Team

Beginning researchers often mistakenly believe this section refers to an exhaustive review of the literature on the research subject. However, the reviewers are actually asking the author to present their own expertise on the research topic along with the expertise of the research team. A discussion of the PI's background, including all previous research projects, publications, and current practice, is foundational.[4,7] This section gives the research team the opportunity to demonstrate to the reviewers that they have the expertise and capability to conduct the proposed research and add strength to their application.[4,7] Another recommendation is to include a summary of the expertise of the provider institution to implement the project, faculty expertise, expertise of team members, and past history of grant funding.[7,8]

Another topic that may be addressed under the "Preliminary Studies" section is any previous experience the research team has with the intended instruments, pilot studies conducted, relevant teaching experience, and membership on task forces or organizations that have provided the team with a perspective on the problem.[7]

When writing for a federal grant, biographical sketches are placed on a form provided within the grant packet. Generally these bio sketches are limited to two pages, which will require the author to highlight specific areas of expertise for participating faculty that relate to the proposed project. This bio sketch must be very specific and very strong to convince the agency that the research team is capable of conducting the research or project.[8]

Methods

The methods section clearly and succinctly describes the plan for conducting the research. Research methods should be explained thoroughly so that the grant reader will have no question of how the study will be conducted[3,7] (see Appendix D). The methods section will vary as to the subcomponents under this section, depending on the research design; however, the following subheadings are offered as a generic standard: (1) research design, (2) a detailed description of the instrumentation, (3) a description of the sampling plan, (4) methods of data production, including any specific procedures, (5) methods of analysis, (6) a detailed time frame that delineates the time each section is expected to be conducted and completed, and (7) discussion of any potential

methodological problems and how these problems will be addressed.[3,7]

Congruency among all sections is essential. There is nothing more frustrating to a reviewer than to read a proposal in which there is little congruency between the problems discussed, rationales or specific aims of the project, and the methods.[7]

Research Design

The most important point in the design is that it is congruent with the stated problem to be studied. A discussion of whether the research project will be an experimental or nonexperimental design is imperative. The PI must also present a discussion of whether the research will utilize a qualitative research design, a quantitative research design, or a triangulated design that incorporates several different designs. Examples of some nonexperimental designs are descriptive research, case studies, surveys (interviews, questionnaires), and record reviews. The classic experimental design utilizes maximum control over as many variables as possible to measure the effect of a proposed causative agent, the independent variable. Partially experimental (quasi experimental) is a common design utilized by many researchers. A quasi-experimental design utilizes variables that are either unable to be completely manipulated or the researcher is unable to directly control the variables. The strongest and most scientifically accepted design is the double-blinded, randomized quantitative experimental design.[1,3,7]

Instruments

All instruments that will be used to conduct the research must be described. A discussion of the reliability and validity of the instruments must be presented. In general, validity lets the reader know that the instrument measures what it is intended to measure, and reliability confirms that the instrument is reliable over repeated uses and over time.[1,3,7] If the instrument has been used in similar research projects, this should also be noted along with the validity and reliability data produced. Include any pilot data that has been generated with the use of the tool.[3] If biomedical instruments are used in the research, a discussion of previous testing results and calibration procedures must be established[3] (see Appendix E).

Finally, a discussion about the proficiency of the researchers in their ability to use the instrumentation correctly needs to be addressed. If there is more than one researcher utilizing the instrument interrater reliability must be documented.[3]

Sample

A description of the target population for the study and the procedures for participant selection is required. Discuss the adequacy of the sample size, remembering that one must fully justify the sample population and size of the sample. Generally, if a quantitative research design is used, a power analysis is required to justify the sample size.[7] A discussion of the inclusion and exclusion criteria and any limitations the sample presents to the study must be included.[3,7,11] Information on how the population will be accessed and supportive documentation that would allow the researchers access to the sample must also be addressed[7] (see Appendix F).

Investigators conducting clinical trials that are seeking government funding must include women, children, and minorities whenever possible. In accordance to the NIH Revitalization Act of 1993, Public Law 103-43, women, minorities, and their subpopulation are to be recruited in all clinical research studies, especially clinical trials. This law ensures that information obtained from the research study will benefit all Americans and not discriminate against gender or cultural biases (see *Federal Register,* 1994, p. 14509 for further information on this topic).[13]

Method of Analysis

The plan for data analysis should include a detailed discussion of the type of data analysis used and the method of analysis. If statistical analyses are to be used, a discussion of the type of statistical analysis should be provided along with the rationale for the analysis[3,7,12] (see Appendix G).

Time Frame

Include a time plan for data production, analysis, interpretation, and preparation of the final report. A detailed time frame for completing each section of the study is recommended.[3] Include flowcharts

and other diagrams highlighting the order and interrelationships of the project activities within the time frame.[7] Time lines also help to serve as a reminder to the PI of what needs to be accomplished by a given deadline and how responsibilities are divided among the research team.[1,7]

Protection of Human Subjects

If the research project involves collection of data from human subjects or animals, then the procedures that will protect the rights of all parties must be included, and one must demonstrate how risks to all subjects will be minimized. All studies involving human or animal subjects must first obtain approval from the institution's Institutional Review Board (IRB) before the research can begin.[7] The researcher must contact the IRB of the institution in which the research will be conducted and submit required forms for the IRB to thoroughly review the study and determine whether or not the researcher has sufficiently protected patients or animals from harm. The study cannot begin until IRB approval is obtained.

Literature Cited

Literature cited represents a complete list of references used in the text of the grant application.[7] These references should reflect current (usually within the past five years), reliable, and valid resources.[1]

Consultants

If consultants will be utilized throughout the conduction of the project, such as statistical analysis, a letter from each consultant and collaborator must be included in the proposal, confirming their willingness to serve on the project.[7]

Appendices

Appendices include all the information that is not in the body of the grant. Some items frequently found in the appendices include curriculum vitae, position descriptions, letters of agreement, agency sponsorship, instruments, sample size estimates, and coding or scoring instructions.[1,4,7,8] These materials may also include proposed letters of consent, letters of cooperation from institutions that will provide access to subjects, complex statistical models, and published papers of the research team.[7]

Budget

Most funding agencies will require a detailed budget for the project. Budgets include personnel salaries, equipment, supplies, and consultant fees. Each section of the budget should include a narrative account to justify the budget amount along with numerical recording for each requested item. The budget must be written so that it is clear and understandable to the reviewer.[8] Personnel costs may include a project director, principle investigators, statisticians, and clerical personnel. The level of time commitment to the project should be spelled out clearly.[11] Equipment that must be purchased may include books, papers for photocopying, stationary, postage, tape recorder, poster productions, or slide production.[11]

Another consideration that needs to be addressed under the budget section is travel time for the research team along with the cost of traveling to and from meetings and conferences. Financial officers of the institution are an invaluable source of support and can offer information on constructing a project budget. Often financial officers will review the proposed budget and calculate wages, personnel benefits, costs for copying, paper, organizational overheads, and so forth.[11]

Finally, the budget should be realistic. If the study will actually require multiple small grants, then request that amount up front. Discuss how the project will move forward if the entire grant request is not awarded.[5]

Putting It All Together

Remember, the most important goal of grant writing is to obtain funding. The proposal should be written in an interesting manner that flows with the project. The project should begin with a sentence that will draw the reader in and keep the reviewers interested throughout. Strict adherence to the published agency guidelines will help direct the flow of the proposal. Tables provide the reviewer with background information, and useful

charts provide a shorthand review of important information. Keep the proposal strong by highlighting the benefits of the project throughout the proposal.

Finally, a cover letter to the agency is always necessary, stating the importance of funding the proposal.[8] The cover letter should demonstrate endorsement of the project by the appropriate board or administration giving authority to the project director, hint at proposal content, and commit to following the letter by a phone call or appointment.[1]

Funding

Because the goal of any research project is to obtain funding, a brief discussion of funding agencies is presented. Basically, there are four types of grants that will receive funding: (1) research, (2) training, (3) arts, and (4) humanities. The money or funding comes from five principle sources: (1) federal, (2) states, (3) foundations, (4) corporations, and (5) individuals. Federal grants may be found in the *Federal Register,* the *Federal Contracts and Grants Weekly,* and the *Commerce Business Daily.* Most of these sites can be found on the Internet or through governmental contacts. The best place to begin is at the federal government's Web page[8] (http://www.khhs.gov). Appendix H lists additional Internet Web sites.

When locating a funding source, it is important to understand the goals of the funding agency and that they are a good match with your proposal.[6] A recommended starting point is to look at the sponsoring agencies' Web page. For the U.S. government, the Bureau of Health Professionals home page at http://www.hrsa.dhhs.gov.bhpr is a good starting point and provides links to nursing or your specific section.[6] It is possible to obtain copies of funded grant applications within many areas of federal funding. This information can be obtained by writing or faxing the Freedom of Information Coordinator for the Department of Health and Human Services to request copies of the funded grant applications.[6]

Conclusion

There is no magic formula for writing a successful grant. The strategies recommended through-out this chapter should give the proposal writer ideas, guidelines, and strategies to enhance the possibility of obtaining grant funding. If the proposed grant is not accepted initially, know that with many agencies as many as 80% of the submitted grants go unfunded, and even those grants that are eventually funded often go back to the writer for multiple revisions before they are finally approved. PIs should not become discouraged, but rather should keep their nose to the grindstone and read the recommendations made by the review panel, change the grant to adhere to the recommendations, and resubmit the grant.[8,9] Often grant funding is not just a matter of experience but how much stick-to-it-iveness the writer has!!

It is also important to keep a sense of humor and humility.[5] Remember, the reviewers are human, too, and can only evaluate the information provided for them.[5,10] Giving the grant reviewers what they want up front and providing a clean and clearly written grant proposal offers the best chance at obtaining funding. Then, remember the old saying, "Be careful what you wish for, it might just come true"!!! Once you receive the grant, then the real exciting work begins.

REFERENCES

1. Forney, D. F., & Evans, W. (1997). Development of a rural oncology nursing conference: Proposal through implementation. *Oncology Nursing Forum, 24*(3), 537–543.
2. Padilla, G. V. (1999). Writing the research proposal. In M. A. Mateo & K. T. Kirchoff (Eds.), *Using and conducting nursing research in the clinical setting* (2nd ed., pp. 289–300). Philadelphia: Saunders.
3. Woods, N. F. (1988). Generating a research proposal. In N. F. Woods & M. Catanzaro (Eds.), *Nursing research: Theory and practice* (pp. 498–529). St. Louis, MO: Mosby.
4. Kachoyeanos, M. K. (1997). Grant writing. *MCN: American Journal of Maternal Child Nursing, 22*(5), 267.
5. Brown, L. P., Meier, P., Spatz, D. L., Spitzer, A., Finkler, S. A., Jacobsen, B.S., et al. (1997). Resubmission of a grand application: Breastfeeding services for LBW infants. *Nursing Research, 46*(2), 119–122.
6. Grey, M. (2000). Top 10 tips for successful grantsmanship. *Research in Nursing and Health, 23*(2), 91–92.
7. Polit, D. F., & Hungler, B. P. (1995). Writing a research proposal. In D. F. Polit & B. P. Hungler (Eds.), *Nursing research: Principles and methods* (6th ed., pp. 671–694). Philadelphia: Lippincott.

8. Hester, S. H. (2000). Strategies for successful grant acquisition. *Journal of the New York State Nurses Association, 31*(1), 22–26. Retrieved December 27, 2002 from http://www.nysna.org/images/pdfs/journal/spg_smr00.pdf

9. Dahlen, R. (2001). Fundamentals of grant writing: Lessons learned from the process. *Nurse Educator, 26*(2), 54–56.

10. Colgan, S. W. (2001). Top drawer. Software reviews: GrantSlam (for Windows). *Computers in Nursing, 19*(4), 139–141.

11. Preparing a proposal for research. (1998, July). *Nursing Times: Clinical Effectiveness*, 25–27.

12. Crain, H. C., & Broome, M. E. (2000). Tool for planning the grant application process. *Nursing Outlook, 48*(6), 288–293.

13. Harden, J. T., & McFarland, G. (2000). Avoiding gender and minority barriers to NIH funding. *Journal of Nursing Scholarship, 32*(1), 83–86.

Appendix A: Title

Trauma Outcome Study: Pilot Study of Brief Alcohol Intervention for Trauma Patients with Positive Alcohol Findings.

Appendix B: Specific Aims

<u>Specific Aims</u>

In a previous study conducted at Loyola University Medical Center looking at the characteristics of trauma recidivists, 33% of trauma patients tested positive for alcohol.[1] Although this fact seems alarming, the reality is that the national average for alcohol-related injury is closer to 40% to 50% of all trauma victims.[2] The relationship of trauma and alcohol has been discussed in public and political venues nationally and internationally; however, studies of interventional techniques to modify alcohol use and their efficacy in the trauma population are scarce. Few of the 39 randomized controlled studies of brief alcohol intervention in the literature focused on patients in the emergency department (ED) or trauma center. Furthermore, these have not been stratified to explore gender or ethnic differences. There is a need for more intervention studies that focus on the treatment of trauma patients demonstrating alcohol use problems. Therefore this proposed pilot investigation will use a randomized control trial design to test the effectiveness of a brief alcohol intervention for trauma patients who screened positive for possible alcohol problems. In addition, Quality of Life (QOL) will be determined because this concept has not been examined in trauma patients suffering from chronic alcohol disease. This study is unique because it would study a brief intervention conducted by a nurse in a population of acutely injured patients. Secondly, it would seek to acquire and evaluate heretofore-uncollected information relating to the effect of a brief alcohol intervention on quality of life. The specific aims of this study therefore are (1) to examine the effectiveness of a brief alcohol intervention provided to trauma patients who screened positive for possible alcohol problems and (2) to examine their perceived QOL before and after the intervention.

Appendix C: Significance

<u>Significance/Background</u>

In the United States, trauma is a disease of the young and the leading cause of death for those under 35 years of age, resulting in a loss of over 2 million life years annually.[3] Approximately 40% of all U.S. traffic fatalities are associated with the use of alcohol,[2,3,4,5] and nearly half of all hospital trauma beds are occupied by patients who were injured while under the influence of alcohol.[4] The risk for traumatic death is 200% to 800% higher among those who abuse alcohol.[5] More specifically, patients with a chronic alcohol problem are five times more likely to die in a motor vehicle crash, 16 times more likely to die in falls, and 10 times more likely to become fire or burn victims.[6,7] This is why impairment caused by alcohol has been termed the leading risk factor for trauma[8] and the most common chronic comorbid condition found in trauma patients.[9] Although these health statistics are alarming, the financial statistics are equally disconcerting. The cost of health care for alcoholism across the United States escalated to approximately $184.6 billion in 1998 alone.[10]

Although the national problems associated with drinking and trauma are well publicized, it is still astonishing to discover that many people operate motor vehicles while highly impaired. The blood alcohol level measured in one study of trauma patients was reported to be more than twice the legal limit for operating a motor vehicle in many states.[8] Alcohol-related injuries are generally associated with greater injury severity, longer hospitalization, and higher health care costs.[11]

Alcohol-related injuries do not respect gender or age boundaries. Women and adolescents have been shown to suffer a significant degree of traumatic injury and chronic alcohol disease. In fact, women have been reported to manifest a greater degree of alcohol-related physical and psychological harm than males. Adolescents represent an increasing proportion of trauma center admissions across the United States.[12,13]

Although these statistics paint a bleak picture of alcohol-related injuries in the United States, a hospital admission for a traumatic injury can represent a unique opportunity for the health care worker to provide an intervention.[5] Often it is the hospitalization that motivates patients to finally deal with their alcohol problem. It is during this "window of opportunity" that health care workers can make a dramatic impact by providing a brief alcohol intervention (BAI).[5,14,15] This is an opportunity to improve not only the health of the patients, but also the health of their family and community, as well as the general society. The use of BAI motivational techniques is intended to assist patients with alcohol use problems to reduce or eliminate their alcohol consumption. BAIs have been reported useful in 36 of the 39 studies published (Appendix XX), and the findings of these studies indicated BAI was effective. Only 2 studies have reported using BAI in the trauma population,[16,17] both demonstrating positive effects of BAI within this population. Randomized controlled trials conducted in a variety of settings have consistently revealed a reduction in alcohol consumption after participating in a brief intervention program.[20] One study of BAI involving 2,000 trauma patients used a brief alcohol intervention technique and reported a decreased rate of alcohol consumption and trauma recidivism approaching 50%.[16]

<u>Recommended Standards</u>

According to the U.S. Preventative Services Task Force,[18] chronic alcoholism among the trauma population should be approached as a public health problem much like risk factor modification for those patients suffering from coronary artery disease (i.e., dietary control, smoking cessation, and routine exercise). They state, "All persons who use alcohol should be informed of the health and injury risks associated with consumption."[18] Another task force composed of members from the National Highway Traffic Safety Administration, the Emergency Nurses Association, and the American College of Emergency Physicians published recommendations in their document, *Developing Best Practices of*

Emergency Care for the Alcohol Impaired Patient.[19] Recommendations from this national conference encourage all physicians and nurses to conduct alcohol screening for all patients and include brief interventions for patients screening positive for chronic alcohol abuse. A second recommendation is for physicians and nurses to actively participate in research on BAI.

There are also current recommendations for trauma centers to identify and treat trauma patients suffering from chronic alcohol disease.[4] This pilot study proposes to examine the effects of BAIs on the population of trauma patients admitted to LUMC.

Research Questions

1. Is the BAI effective among the trauma population as measured by a change in baseline alcohol consumption?
2. Is the behavior change sustained over time, as measured at one-, three-, and six-month intervals?
3. Do subjects' perceptions of their QOL improve after the brief alcohol intervention?
4. What factors are predictive of BAI success?
5. Are there demonstrable differences between gender or ethnic groups with regard to the effects of BAI on subjects with alcohol use problems and QOL?

Appendix D: Design

<u>Methodology</u>

This pilot study uses a prospective experimental design in which eligible participants are randomly assigned to either a treatment or a control group. Identifying the treatment population is of paramount importance in beginning a study of trauma patients with a possible alcohol disorder. Because laboratory tests are not highly predictive of current alcohol dependence, studies conclude that a combination of blood alcohol tests and interview screens provide the best screening tools in this patient population.[16] Therefore, to determine eligibility for the randomized pilot study, two screening tools will be utilized: (1) the Alcohol Use Disorders Identification Test (AUDIT) (Appendix XX) and (2) the admission blood alcohol level (BAL).

After assignment, all subjects will complete a QOL (SF-12) questionnaire.

Chart data will also be collected on all eligible individuals and will include the following: demographic data, injury severity score, type and intent of injury, previous traumatic injuries, drug and alcohol use, BAL, and drug screen results (Appendix XX).

The control group will receive standard care for the trauma patient and customary alcohol referral. The treatment group will receive standard care, customary alcohol referral, and a BAI. The BAI will last 5 to 30 minutes and be given to the subjects at a time appropriate in their hospital course and at a place convenient to them. The intervention subjects will also be given a handout with references for decreasing alcohol intake (Appendix XX).

Both groups will be contacted by telephone at one, three and six months after hospital release and asked the questions from the AUDIT tool and the SF-12. It is expected that each phone call will take approximately 10 minutes. The treatment group will also receive a follow-up letter reviewing the contents of the BAI. The study design is listed following.

Table D-1. Study Calendar

Method	Interview	Interview	Phone	Phone	Phone
Time	Screening (≥ 8 hours after admission)	Positive screening test (+ AUDIT or BAL)	1 month	3 month	6 month
All trauma pts	AUDIT BAL				
Control	Demographic data	Standard alcohol tx SF-12	AUDIT SF-12	AUDIT SF-12	AUDIT SF-12
Intervention group	Demographic data	Standard alcohol tx SF-12 BAI	Letter AUDIT SF-12	AUDIT SF-12	AUDIT SF-12

<u>Brief Alcohol Intervention</u>

The success of BAI is based on two principles: (1) the patient is assessed for readiness to change; the intervention is then modified based on the patient's readiness to change; and (2) a brief intervention should be conducted as a motivational interview. The focus should be on motivating the patient to change and not to simply advise the patient.

The PI, a nurse practitioner who has had training in conducting motivational interviewing, will conduct the BAI interview. The motivational interview training consists of viewing eight hours of videotapes

produced by the motivational interview experts, Miller and Rollnick, and knowledge of the information provided by two motivational interviewing books written by the same authors.[26,27]

Once the patient's severity of alcohol use is determined (Appendix XX), then the patient will be evaluated according to his or her readiness to change. Readiness to change is measured using a tool developed by Prochaska and DiClemente[28] (Appendix XX). The first stage on the continuum of readiness to change is precontemplation. In the precontemplation stage, the patient does not see his or her alcohol intake as a problem and is not considering change. The second stage is the contemplation stage, whereby the patients believe that alcohol could be a problem in their lives but are ambivalent to change. The third stage is action, in which the patient is ready for action soon or has already started to take action to change. According to Rollnick, Mason, and Butler,[29] two additional components that influence the patient's readiness to change include the importance of the subject and the confidence that he or she could be successful. Depending on where the patient is on the readiness to change continuum determines the type of BAI implemented.

The BAI to be used in this study uses the FRAMES model (Appendix XX) developed by Bein et al.[20] The FRAMES model represents six steps of successful brief interventions: (1) feedback, (2) responsibility, (3) advice, (4) menu, (5) empathy, and (6) self-efficacy. Following is a guide for a BAI proposed for use in this study.

1. Determine whether the patient represents a hazardous or harmful drinker (Appendix XX).
2. Know the stages of change and determine whether or not the patient is ready for the intervention (Appendix XX).
3. Administer the six major components of effective interventions (Appendix XX): FRAMES
   a. Feedback: Respectfully give specific information that concerns the patient.
   b. Responsibility: Stress that the patient is responsible for any change.
   c. Advice: Respectfully give advice to the patient.
   d. Menu: Offer patient a menu of choices.
   e. Empathy: Listen and respond with accurate reflective statements.
   f. Self-efficacy: (1) Change is possible, and (2) change is beneficial.

During the feedback phase, the patients will be given the results of the data obtained from the assessment and the current standards for alcohol use in the United States. The patients will be advised of how they compare to the acceptable low-risk drinking standards as outlined by the National Institution on Alcohol Abuse and Alcoholism.[30] Patients are then motivated to assume responsibility for their choice to change in a respectful manner. Advice to patients depends on their readiness to change. If patients are not ready to change, simply raising awareness of their situation and questioning their interpretation of their problem may be enough to move them to the contemplation and action stage. If the patients are in the contemplative stage, the feedback could move them to the action stage. If the patients are in the action stage, then they would be given tips to cut down on their drinking. A booklet of handouts printed with permission from the National Institute on Alcohol Abuse and Alcoholism[30] (Appendix XX) on drinking and how to cut down on drinking and available support groups will be provided to all patients in the treatment group. Patients are given empathy in their current situation, and the interviewer recognizes that change is difficult. Finally, in promoting self-efficacy, the interviewer supports the patients in their desire to change and reinforces the knowledge that change is possible and even beneficial.

Follow-up

Participants in the intervention group will receive a summary letter one month postdischarge outlining the intervention discussed. All participants will be contacted by phone at one, three, and six months postdischarge, asked to repeat the AUDIT and SF-12 tools, and asked if they have had any repeat injuries or citations for drinking and driving.

Appendix E: Instruments

After examining available screening tools, the AUDIT test gives the most information being sought in this study, namely amount and frequency of alcohol intake, allows for easy scoring into risk stratification, takes approximately 10 to 20 minutes to administer, and has reported sensitivity of .75 and specificity of .89[22] (Appendix XX).

The QOL tool that will be used is the General Health Screening Questionnaire, the SF-12 (Appendix XX). This tool has demonstrated reliability and validity scores of .89 and .86, respectively.[24] The tool elicits a health profile using 12 questions that focus on health-related QOL. It takes approximately two minutes to administer and will offer valuable insight on the patient's quality of life. This test can be self-administered; however, the PI will assist patients if they are having difficulty with the questions.

Appendix F: Sample

After IRB approval is received, all trauma patients who are ≥18 years old, are English speaking, do not have a severe head injury (Glasgow Coma Scale score ≥14), and are medically stable enough to complete an interview will be approached to determine eligibility for participation and to obtain informed consent. This will not occur until at least eight or more hours after admission to ensure that patients are not intoxicated while obtaining informed consent or during the screening test.

All patients who test positive for either the presence of alcohol in their blood (any value) or alcohol use disorder problems (score of eight or more) will be eligible for the intervention study. A sample size of 50 subjects is requested (25 to each group). A pilot of 50 subjects was determined suitable based on a review of the current literature and the number of variables to be examined.

Eligible participants will be randomly assigned to the treatment or control group. This will be determined by pulling from an envelope a piece of paper marked "control" or "treatment."

Appendix G: Method of Analysis

Frequency distributions will be used to describe demographic characteristics. Repeated measures of analysis of variance will evaluate changes in alcohol use and QOL over time. Chi-square test will be used to evaluate demographic differences related to gender and ethnicity. Logistic regression will be used to evaluate factors associated with positive response to BAI.

Appendix H: Web Sites for Possible Funding Sources[1,8,13]

http//www.ena.org	Emergency Nurses Association
http://www.mindspring.com/~ajgrant/guide.htm	A Grant Seekers Guide to the Internet: Reviewed and Revisited
http://fdncenter.org	The Foundation Center
http://www.tgci.com	Grantmanship Center
http://www.hhs.gov	U.S. Department of Health and Human Services
http://www.hrsa.gov	Health Resources and Services Administration (HRSA)
http://cbdnet.access.gpo.gov	Commerce Business Daily
http://www.mchb.hrsa.gov	HRSA Maternal & Child Health Bureau
http://www.nih.gov	National Institutes of Health
http://www.ahcpr.gov	Agency for Healthcare Research & Quality
http://www.cdc.gov	Centers for Disease Control
http://www.va.gov	Department of Veterans Affairs
http://www.yahoo.com	Search engine
http://www.altavista.com	Search engine
http://www.google.com	Search engine
http://www.medtrib.com	The Medical Tribune
http://www.cancer.org	American Cancer Society
http://www.americanheart.org	American Heart Association
http://www.diabetes.org	American Diabetes Foundation
http://www.rwjf.org	Robert Woods Johnson Foundation

19 COLLABORATIVE PRACTICE AGREEMENTS

Karen Sue Hoyt, RN, MN, PhD(c), CEN

Collaborative practice agreements are often at the center of the advanced practice nurse's (APN) contract and are often the one legal document that allows APNs to practice in an independent or semi-independent role. Many states require collaborative practice agreements between APNs and physicians for them to legally practice and obtain reimbursement. Therefore it is important for APNs to have a thorough understanding of collaborative practice agreements and the underlying ramifications for practice.

Definitions of Collaboration

Merriam-Webster's Collegiate Dictionary defines *collaboration* as "the ability to work jointly with others or together especially in an intellectual endeavor; to cooperate with an agency or instrumentality with which one is not immediately connected."[1] According to Siegler and Messett, the definition of collaboration in health care can be "academic, strategic, or statutory."[2] There are also several organizational and institutional definitions that can assist one in interpreting what collaboration means within the context of health care.

The document *Scope of Practice Document for the Nurse Practitioner in the Emergency Care Setting*[3] emphasizes that there should be "an emphasis on collaborative practice. . . ." Furthermore, the Emergency Nurses Association (ENA) supports collaboration between APNs and physicians and offers this collaboration as a possible solution to the health care crisis facing the nation today. The ENA's position statement on advanced practice nursing states that clinical nurse specialists (CNSs) and nurse practitioners (NPs) have been established as APNs since 1965. Not only are these nurses seen as clinical patient care experts, but also expanded roles of APNs involve leadership, administration, consultation, education, and research.[4] In the position statement, the rationale supporting APNs in the emergency department (ED) comes from the need for cost-effective and creative approaches to the care of the ED patient. The APN is uniquely prepared and positioned to provide this collaborative care to achieve better patient outcomes.

APN organizations also discuss collaboration. The American Academy of Nurse Practitioners (AANP), for example, states that APNs make both independent and collaborative decisions regarding the health of patients.[5] The National Association of Clinical Nurse Specialists (NACNS) views the three spheres of CNS influence as necessitating interdisciplinary collaboration; the CNS must possess knowledge and skill competencies to become an effective collaborator.[6]

The American Nurses Association (ANA) defines collaboration as "a partnership in which the power among the partners is valued by each party and in which there is recognition and acceptance of separate and combined spheres of activity and responsibility, mutual safeguarding of the legitimate interests of each party, and a community of goals."[7]

The joint task force of the ANA and the American Medical Association (AMA) relates that collaboration is a process in which both physicians and nurses plan and practice together collegially and work independently within the boundaries of their scope of practice. Physicians and nurses provide collaboration through the values they share. This collaboration is performed with mutual acknowledgment and respect for each other's contribution to the care of patients, their families, and their community.[2]

The American Academy of Emergency Medicine's (AAEM) position statement on physician assistants (PAs) and NPs takes a different approach to collaboration. AAEM believes patients should have access to a physician board certified in emergency medicine and therefore opposes off-site supervision of PAs and NPs in EDs.[8] Though the American College of Emergency Physicians (ACEP) has developed guidelines on the role of APNs (i.e., NPs) in the ED, there is no mention of instituting collaborative practice agreements.[9] ACEP does state that "NPs should work clinically with the supervision of an emergency physician who is present in the ED or available for consultation."[9]

A final definition of collaboration is one that is used by federal agencies with regard to reimbursement for an APN (i.e., an NP). For instance, to be eligible for government reimbursement, that definition of collaboration is "a process in which an NP works with a physician to deliver health care services within the scope of the NP's professional expertise, with medical direction and appropriate supervision as provided for in jointly developed guidelines or other mechanisms as defined by the law of the state in which services are performed."[2]

Resurgence of APNs

There has been an explosion of APNs in the United States over the last few decades. There are nearly 60,000 CNSs in the United States according to the NACNS, and NPs have jumped from about 30,000 to over 65,000 in just 10 years.[6] By 2005, it is projected that there will be more than 100,000 NPs in the country.[5] Currently 34 states have allowed NPs to practice collaboratively, and most (85%) NPs practice in ambulatory settings. AANP also purports there is nothing in the law mandating NPs have daily encounters with physicians, and each situation is practice dependent. In some states written practice agreements with physicians that clarify the collaboration plan are required.[5]

Programs for emergency nurse practitioners (ENPs) are also emerging. In one program, the job description of the ENP recognizes that ". . . the ENP functions as a member of an interdisciplinary team offering health care to patients who

seek ED services. The ENP also serves as a part of a collaborative team which is comprised of physicians, nurses, and other health care personnel. The emergency nurse practitioner has a sponsoring physician who supervisors the ENP and depending on whether or not the practitioner and the institution agree to a dependent or independent practice, the role of this supervising physician varies. The ENP will meet all rules and regulations of their state nursing board and of their institution's bylaws."[3] In other words, all policies and procedures outlined for ENPs will be followed if the ENP is in an independent practice. The supervising physician and nurse practitioner will mutually develop protocols utilized by the ENP to provide services to ED patients. The ENP having prescriptive authority will also follow guidelines for writing prescriptions based on the regulations by their board of nursing and/or medical examiners.[10]

Barriers to Collaboration

Traditional barriers to collaboration have always had to do with practice autonomy, prescriptive authority, reimbursement, and provider status. NPs and physicians, as one example, are now employed in similar practices in which their skills and competencies complement each other.[11] Turf wars regarding the scope of practice of APNs have also obstructed collaboration. Presently, APNs have had to overcome many barriers to the implementation of collaborative practice agreements because only 21 states and the District of Columbia allow some degree of independent practice for NPs, for example. Currently, the remaining states, however, require some degree of physician collaboration. Because the legal status and regulation of NPs varies significantly from state to state, the relationship of medical doctors (MDs) and NPs has been jeopardized, although many NPs and physicians embrace collegiality. Therefore, barriers to independent practice for APNs will continue to make collaborative efforts more difficult between MDs and NPs.[12]

The ongoing debate regarding collaboration between physicians and nurses, particularly NPs, has been shaped by many forces. The major forces that actually brought about the inception of collaboration were a result of the lack of health

insurance coverage in the United States; the introduction of managed care plans, which commenced in the 1980s; and the many increased opportunities for APNs in the Unites States (i.e., more programs, changing regulations, and an emphasis on health promotion, disease prevention, and a holistic approach to care). These factors were the catalysts that made physicians and other health care providers entertain the idea of collaboration with NPs.[12]

There are arguments for and against separate APN roles between not only physicians and APNs (e.g., NPs), but between NPs and CNSs. According to Conger, an argument has been put forth for separate advanced practice roles between the CNS/case manager role and the NP role using a model that depicts these roles as separate and distinct. It is through this "separate collaboration" that the patient is offered more efficient, more cost effective, and higher quality care.[13]

Collaborative Practice Arrangements

Traditionally, the AMA supports collaborative arrangements with nonphysicians rather than independent practice and wholeheartedly supports collaborative practice among NPs. Many physicians are now hiring NPs into their practices or making them part of their teams in hospital institutions.[12]

Advanced practice arrangements are changing day to day in several states. Some states mandate that NPs practice with a physician, using protocols or guidelines to direct patient care. This is considered a more traditional, dependent role. Other states, however, allow the NP to practice more collegially with the physician. Thus, the NP has a very independent role.[3]

Some arrangements are also based on location of employment and practice models. For example, NPs in the ED have been able to provide more comprehensive health care to patients. Ramos explained that when the physician practice includes an NP, this collaboration between the NP and the MD also improves the quality of care.[14] It may also influence utilization rates. In a study on effective clinical practice in which a comparison of

resource utilization in NPs and physicians was performed, Hemani, Rastegar, Hill, and al-Ibrahim indicated resource utilization for patients assigned to an NP was higher than that for patients assigned to a resident or an attending physician.[15]

Models of advanced nursing practice have even been jointly funded through nursing and medicine in the past decade. For example, a model at Children's Hospital in Philadelphia was developed utilizing a matrix reporting structure with a CNS reporting concurrently to both a nursing director and a physician. By using such a model, the authors reported clinical benefits not only to the patients and their families but also to provider satisfaction of the APN, physician, institution, and staff members.[16]

Collaboration between APNs and MDs offers unique services to patients. Most physicians who hire NPs, for example, state that working collaboratively frees the MD up to actually see more patients—patients who need the MD the most.[11]

Collaboration also means different things to different groups. For instance, physicians in New York learned the value of collaboration nearly 20 years ago by hiring NPs into their practice. As a result of hiring NPs in what is now a primary care practice, the practice is able to see more patients and provide more cost-effective care. As one physician in the group stated, "What makes this practice particularly unusual is that the nurse practitioners maintain their own patient panels. Their relationship with the physician is one of collaboration—a mode of practice that has been the subject of heated debate elsewhere." NPs consult with MDs when they have questions or require consultation. In another article by the same author, it was noted that government agencies also showed that NPs provide excellent primary care. In an important Gallup Poll conducted in 1993, consumers were willing to see an NP 86% of the time.[11]

Changing Roles: Collaborative Practice Agreements

The role of the APN lends itself, at times, to ambiguity and confusion because APNs "define" themselves differently. According to Redekopp,[17]

role confusion may result in frustration and may lead to barriers to collaboration. Because there are several different roles for the APN (i.e., NP, CNS), role confusion also can contribute to conflict, which prevents the APN from optimizing knowledge and skills.[18] At times this has even brought about the deletion of the advanced practice position in various institutions. Furthermore, a myriad of factors influencing the delineation of the role has included (1) the ever-changing needs of patients, (2) the needs of the families of these patients, (3) interdisciplinary team members, (4) health care institutions, and (5) community agencies. Additionally, the knowledge, skills, and experiences of the APN also play a major part in role clarification.[6] To avoid role confusion, APNs need to clearly delineate their role to others. One way to do this is for the APN and others (i.e., physician), working in collaboration, to write a collaborative practice agreement.[18]

A collaborative practice agreement is considered a legal document and should be clearly understood by all parties before the agreement is signed. There are several components to the collaborative practice agreement that are standard. The introduction should identify the parties involved and the facility of practice. There must be a clear requirement for education and training. Prescriptive authority should be delineated so all parties know the boundaries of authority. A clear chain of command should be written under the section entitled "Supervision and Consultation." The duties and expectations of the APN should be described, and it should be very clear in the contract when supervision, physician consultation, or referrals are required. Examples of consultation should be provided for clarification. Documentation requirements should also be included as well as how the protocols are approved and how the care of the patients is evaluated. A sample collaborative practice agreement is provided in Appendix A.

Summary

In summary, in recent years, APNs have begun to work more collegially with physicians, other APNs, and other agencies to improve the health care system. Through collaboration with others, APNs can more fully meet the goals and objectives of the patient while realizing a more satisfying practice environment. Evidence has shown that collaborative practice agreements "that work" improve not only the health outcomes of patients but also the lives of those who practice in them.

REFERENCES

1. *Merriam-Webster dictionary online.* (n.d.). Retrieved June 2, 2002, from http://www.m-w.com
2. Siegler, E. L., & Messett, E. (2000). Nurse practitioners and physician assistants in the health care system. *Annals of Long-Term Care: Clinical Care and Aging, 8*(Special Issue), 56–57.
3. Cole, F. L., Ramirez, E., & Luna-Gonzales, H. (1999). *Scope of practice for the nurse practitioner in the emergency care setting.* Des Plaines, IL: Emergency Nurses Association.
4. Emergency Nurse Association. (2000). *Advanced practice in emergency nursing* [Position statement]. Des Plaines, IL: Author.
5. American Academy of Nurse Practitioners. (2002). *Nurse practitioner as an advanced practice nurse* [Role position statement]. Retrieved June 2, 2002 from http://www.aanp.org/np_advanced_practice.htm
6. National Association of Clinical Nurse Specialists. (1998). *Statement on clinical nurse specialist practice and education.* Harrisburg, PA: Author.
7. American Nurses Association. (1995). *Nursing: A social policy statement.* Kansas City, MO: Author.
8. American Academy of Emergency Medicine. (2000). *Position statement on physician assistants/nurse practitioners.* Retrieved March 5, 2002 from http://www.aaem.org/positionstatements/physicianasst.shtml
9. American College of Emergency Physicians. (2000). *Guidelines on the role of nurse practitioners in the emergency department* [Policy statement]. Retrieved June 2, 2002 from http://www.acep.org/1,583,0.html
10. Ramirez, E. (1996). A personal perspective: Nurse practitioner in the emergency department. *Journal of Emergency Nursing, 22*(6), 538–540.
11. Flanagan, L. (1998). Nurse practitioners: Growing competition for family physicians? *Family Practice Management, 5*(9). Retrieved March 5, 2002 from http://www.aafp.org/fpm/981000fm/nurse.html
12. Greene, J. (2001, March 12). Growing ranks: Benefits of collaboration with nurse practitioners. *Amednews.com.* Retrieved March 5, 2001 from http://www.ama-assn.org/sci-pubs/amnews/pick_01/prsa0312.htm
13. Conger, M., & Craig, C. (1998). Advanced nurse practice. A model for collaboration. *Nursing Case Management, 3*(3), 120–127.
14. Ramos, L. (n.d.). *Nurse practitioners extend health care's reach.* Retrieved March 5, 2002 from http://www.rush.edu/professionals/nursing/article.html

15. Hemani, A., Rastegar, D. A., Hill, C., & al-Ibrahim, M. S. (1999). A comparison of resource utilization in nurse practitioners and physicians [Electronic version]. *Effective Clinical Practice, 2*(6), 258–265. Retrieved June 2, 2002 from http://www.acponline.org/journals/ecp/novdec99/hemani.htm

16. Verger, J. (2002). *Advanced practice nursing in pediatric critical care*. Retrieved June 2, 2002 from http://pedsccm.wustl.edu/NURSING/APN_info.html

17. Redekopp, M. A. (1997). Clinical nurse specialist role confusion: The need for identity. *Clinical Nurse Specialist, 11*(2), 87–91.

18. Longworth, J. C. (2001). *Collaborative practice agreement*. Retrieved March 5, 2002 from http://www.nonpf.com/fpcollabagreesample.htm

Appendix A
Sample Collaborative Practice Agreement

A sample collaborative practice agreement is listed herein. The example used is that of the advanced practice role of the NP.

Introduction

The purpose of this document is to permit nurse practitioner _____(name of NP)_____ at _____(facility)_____ to see clients and practice under the attached protocols without the direct supervision of _____(name of MD)_____, as specified in the _____(State Medical Practice Act)_____. This information also contains a guide to collaboration between the supervising physician and the nurse practitioners.

Education and Training

The nurse practitioner and the physician must possess a current, valid license from the licensing board in their state.

Prescriptive Authority

The nurse practitioner listed herein is authorized to prescribe medications (excluding controlled substances) as authorized by _____(State Board of Registered Nursing)_____. This authority shall be delegated by the _____(Medical Director of Named Institution)_____ as indicated in _____(Medical Staff Policy)_____. It is the responsibility of the nurse practitioner to obtain a furnishing number and drug enforcement agency (DEA) number from their State Board of Nursing. The Medical Director of said institution shall notify their State Board of Medical Examiners, in writing, of their intent to delegate this prescriptive authority to the nurse practitioner. Prescription references will be the most current Physician's Desk Reference (or other approved sources), and restrictions may be placed on the prescribing of medications according to approved institutional formularies.

Supervision and Consultation

Nurse practitioners practice independently under the established protocols of _____(Name of Institution)_____. The nurse practitioner is required to provide health services to patients (at said agency). Services the nurse practitioner will provide include: (a) health promotion and screening, (b) management of acute, episodic illness and injury, and (c) management of chronic illnesses considered stable. All other patients will be referred to the appropriate health care provider.

Consultation with the supervising physician or another physician designee is available 24 hours per day, 7 days per week on-site or via phone. Consultation is recommended and is encouraged whenever the nurse practitioner has questions about a patient. Consultation is required for any condition outside the scope of practice of the nurse practitioner as determined by the protocols that have been set forth. If physician–nurse practitioner consultation occurs, written documentation to that effect will be noted in the medical record of the patient within 24 hours.

Consultative examples, include, but are not limited to (a) conditions where the patient fails to respond to a set regimen of care, (b) unstable acute illnesses or injuries, (c) unstable chronic illnesses or injuries, (d) any diagnosis or treatment that is not listed in the established protocols, and (e) any time a patient refuses care by a nurse practitioner or requests to be seen by a physician.

Patient Documentation

Nurse practitioners and physicians are required to provide complete, legible, written or dictated documentation using the subjective, objective, assessment, and plan (SOAP) format.

Approval Process

The protocols and this agreement will be revised and approved on an annual basis from the initial signing date. It is the responsibility of the medical director to ensure that written approval is obtained from the supervising physician, other physicians, and nurse practitioners by that date.

Care Evaluation

The evaluation of clinical care will be performed on a minimum of 20% of the nurse practitioner's charts by the supervising physician. During the probationary six-month period, the nurse practitioner can be terminated at any time. After that time, an annual review will be done. The Quality Improvement Committee of the Department will also provide periodic review of both physician and nurse practitioner charts.

Collaboration Agreement: Signatures

I (we) agree to the terms set forth in this collaborative practice agreement.

Date _____ Print Name _____ Signature _____
                Medical Director

Date _____ Print Name _____ Signature _____
                Supervising Physician

Date _____ Print Name _____ Signature _____
                Supervising Nurse Practitioner

Date _____ Print Name _____ Signature _____
                Nurse Practitioner

20 CERTIFICATION

Darcy Egging, RN, MS, CS-ANP, CEN

Advanced practice nurses (APNs) need certification to guarantee minimum competencies within their area of expertise. The history of certification began within medical societies; however, it was not until the 1940s that the American Association of Nurse Anesthetists introduced the first nursing certification. In 1974 the American Nurses Association developed a formal recognition of achievement of performance and education via certification. Since that time, there has been an explosion in the numbers and types of certification examinations given by a variety of organizations.[1,2] This explosion may be an indirect response to the regulation of advanced practice nursing. The purpose of this chapter is to explore what certification is, why it is important, and how it affects APNs in emergency departments (EDs).

Forms of Regulation

Regulation of a profession falls into one of four levels: (1) certification, (2) licensure, (3) registration, and (4) designation. This chapter will focus on the first three forms.[1,3]

Certification is defined as a process by which a nongovernmental agency or association has assessed that a person has met certain predetermined criteria ensuring that the APN has demonstrated the minimum skills necessary to practice in a particular specialty.[4,5,6] Professional certification, as defined by the American Nurses Credentialing Center (ANCC), is based on predetermined standards and validates a registered nurse's (RN's) qualifications, knowledge, and practice in a defined functional or clinical area of nursing.[6] The National Organization for Competency Assurance (NOCA) defines certification as a way to recognize an individual for advanced knowledge and skill.[7] Through certification, the knowledge

needed for safe and proficient care is measured.[8] Although the original intent of certification was voluntary, many states now require APNs to take and pass a national examination as a part of their license requirement.[9,10]

Licensure defines the scope and sets the boundaries of practice for the APN. Licensure resides within state law. State law takes two forms, statutes and regulations (rules); it is important to understand the difference between these laws. Statute law is made by the legislature, whereas regulations are made by state agencies under the executive branch. Regulations cannot contradict statutes; usually they explain the statute to assist government administration.[11]

When one wants to change a statute, the support of a legislator is required for the bill to be introduced. If, however, there were a need to change a regulation, one would either have to enlist the support of the state agency or convince a legislator to introduce a bill that would override the regulation.[11]

When regulatory changes are proposed, an official notification needs to be filed within a given period of time for public comment. Once the proposed regulation becomes final, the law is then republished in final form in the state's register. Much of the state law that governs APN practice appears in regulation form.[11] Licensure enables states to take disciplinary action against inferior practice. Additionally licensure allows for title protection, which prohibits the use of a professional designation by someone who has not met the appropriate criteria.[1]

Registration is simply a list in the state's records of the names of individuals, such as nurses, who have obtained licensure. Registration does not

ensure competency nor does it define practice.[12] This is the least restrictive form of regulation.[7]

All three forms of regulation described earlier allow for title protection. Certification and licensure imply title protection. Only those who have successfully passed the certification can use the title. When speaking of licensure, only those individuals who hold the license may use the title. Registration, on the other hand, allows title protection by applying to a governmental agency.[7]

Licensure of Professional Nursing

Virtually every state has developed some form of regulation for advanced nursing practice that requires passage of a certification examination. In many states the reference to passing a nationally recognized certification has been placed into statutory law. Thus certifying organizations must ensure that their examinations are psychometrically sound and legally defensible for these regulatory purposes. For example, the National Council of State Boards of Nursing (NCSBN) identified the criteria for regulatory sufficiency for certification examinations to include: a design geared toward entry-level competencies, exclusively job-related knowledge and skills, pass/fail at the point of the minimum-essential level for safety and effectiveness, and use of generally accepted testing practices.[13] Therefore, the purpose of these certification examinations is to measure competence in the essential functions of the profession.[14]

The NCSBN published a position paper that addressed the responsibilities of regulation regarding APN practice. This paper states that the foremost responsibility of nursing regulation is the protection of health, safety, and welfare. The goal is to identify essential qualifications for APN licensure and to evaluate whether the individual has met those qualifications. Because regulation may prohibit entry into advanced nursing practice, there needs to be consideration given to the possibility of a legal challenge. It is important, therefore, that regulations balance restrictions to practice with public safety.[14] The NCSBN can only make proposals to the state boards of nursing; it cannot enact the proposal into law.[15] It is the board of nursing in each state, under the authority of the Nursing Practice Act, that establishes statutory authority for licensure of RNs and APNs, which includes the use of a title, scope of practice, standards of practice, and a disciplinary process.[13]

Why is this important for the APN who is practicing in the ED? It is important because currently there is no certification specifically addressing the body of knowledge that is needed to practice in the ED. APNs have additional education and experience, and therefore they function with more autonomy and independence. Nurse practitioners (NPs) and clinical nurse specialists (CNSs) each have a specific scope of practice with some overlapping functions. The legal scope of practice reflects the uniqueness of the role. Because of this uniqueness, it is difficult for an organization such as Board of Certification for Emergency Nursing (BCEN) to develop a universal test that meets both the NP and CNS scopes of practice in one broad examination. The purpose of certification in emergency nursing (CEN®) is to provide a mechanism to regularly measure the attainment and simulated application of a defined body of emergency nursing knowledge needed to function at the *competent* level, according to BCEN.[16] Because there is not a specific examination for APNs in the ED, some of our colleagues may have a difficult time obtaining employment in this arena because of state regulations.

Certification Process

In 2000, the NCSBN convened a task force to make recommendations about APN practice requirements. From this task force, the Uniform Advanced Practice Registered Nurse Licensure/ Authority to Practice Requirements was developed. There are specific requirements for the APN regarding education. The NCSBN criteria for certification programs state that the APN should graduate from a formal graduate advanced practice program with a concentration in the advanced practice specialty for which the APN will be certifying. The program must have both didactic and clinical components. Both direct and indirect clinical supervision should be congruent with the certification and accreditation guidelines for a minimum of 500 clinical hours. With the proliferation of NP programs,[14] it is very important for students looking at programs to know exactly

what examination they will be able to take on graduation.

The core NP examinations are acute care, adult, family, gerontological, pediatric, family psychiatric and mental health, and adult psychiatric and mental health. Core CNS examinations are adult psychiatric and mental health, child or adolescent psychiatric and mental health, community health, gerontological, home health, medical-surgical, and pediatric. The NCSBN task force has expressed concern that many areas of advanced practice have certification examinations, with an expanding area of subspecialty programs, for example CRRN—A (certified rehabilitation registered nurse—advanced). Additional concerns the task force had were

- How to regulate subspecialty APNs within their scope of practice
- Low numbers of candidates, which makes it much harder to develop a valid and reliable exam; therefore, the test may not be psychometrically sound[17]

This task force went on to recommend that the APN should have a broad preparation and that subspecialty credentialing could be attained after first obtaining the minimum entry requirements. Although a generic test has been discussed, there are no current plans to pursue this avenue because of the cost of performing a role delineation study.

The NCSBN task force worked closely with certifying organizations to develop a standard and a process for external review of the certification process. The 2002 recommendations for examinations are listed in Table 20-1.[14]

It is important to note that the current CEN examination does not meet the preceding requirements. When obtaining the designation of CEN, it measures minimal competence level of the staff ED nurse, which is different from the criteria used by state governments to grant legal authority to practice. The CEN examination is not considered an advanced practice examination. The certifying organizations that are routinely accepted by states to meet the requirements for APN national certification are outlined in Table 20-2.

Table 20-1
2002 NCSBN Recommendations for Examinations

1. The scope of credentialing is national.
2. Conditions for taking the examination are consistent with acceptable standards for testing.
3. Educational requirements are consistent with the requirements of the advanced practice specialty.
4. A logical job analysis exists.
5. The examination represents entry-level practice.
6. The examination represents the knowledge, skills, and abilities essential for the delivery of safe and effective advanced nursing care to clients.
7. Examination items are reviewed for content validity, cultural bias, and correct scoring using an established mechanism.
8. Examination items are evaluated for psychometric performance.
9. The passing standard is established using acceptable psychometric standards.
10. Examination security is maintained through established procedures.
11. Certification is issued based on passing the examination and meeting all other certification requirements.
12. A retake policy exists.
13. Certifications maintenance, which includes review of qualifications and continued competence, is in place.
14. Mechanisms are in place for communication to boards of nursing for timely verification of an individual's certification status.
15. An evaluation process is in place to provide quality assurance.

It is very important for APNs to check with the state in which they wish to practice to ascertain what is accepted as a national certification because each state has a different requirement for the certification standard.[3,6] The APN, after successful completion of the certification examination, will be allowed to utilize the credentials bestowed by the certifying organization (i.e., ANP-C).

Issues

Some of the issues revolving around certification include lack of standards for state licensure, titling, and educational requirements. Additionally, for APNs who practice in the ED, there is no set of standards of practice nor is there a specific examination to validate the knowledge needed to practice as an APN in the ED.

Table 20-2	
Certifying Organizations	
CERTIFYING ORGANIZATION	ADVANCED PRACTICE CERTIFICATIONS OFFERED
ANCC	■ Acute Care Nurse Practitioner ■ Adult Nurse Practitioner ■ Family Nurse Practitioner ■ Gerontological Nurse Practitioner ■ Pediatric Nurse Practitioner ■ Adult Psychiatric and Mental Health Nurse Practitioner ■ Family Psychiatric and Mental Health Nurse Practitioner ■ Clinical Specialist in Gerontological Nursing ■ Clinical Specialist in Medical-Surgical Nursing ■ Clinical Specialist in Pediatric Nursing ■ Clinical Specialist in Adult Psychiatric and Mental Health Nursing ■ Clinical Specialist in Child and Adolescent Psychiatric and Mental Health Nursing
AANP (American Academy of Nurse Practitioners)	■ Adult Nurse Practitioner ■ Family Nurse Practitioner
NCC (National Certification Corporation—Neonatal and OB)	■ Women's Health Care Nurse Practitioner ■ Neonatal Care Nurse Practitioner
NCBPNP/N (National Certification Board PNP)	■ Certified Pediatric Nurse Practitioner ■ Currently looking at an Acute Care Pediatric Nurse Practitioner exam
A-ONC (Oncology)	■ Advance Oncology Certified Nurses (does not differentiate between NP or CNS)
ACNM (American College of Nurse Midwives) certification council	■ Certified Nurse Midwife (CNM)

The Pew Health Professions Commission report, entitled *Reforming Health Care Workforce Regulation: Policy Considerations for the 21st Century,* made 10 recommendations for reform of the current regulatory system for health care. There has been much debate about these recommendations from various organizations. The 10 recommendations are listed in Table 20-3.

Although the Pew report does not specifically address APN practice, both the Pew report and the NCSBN *Uniform Advanced Practice Registered Nurse License/Authority to Practice Requirement* paper ask for uniformity in regulatory language. Additionally they both agree that standards need to be set for entry into practice, which includes educational requirements. Although there is disagreement on how this could occur, most agree that this would be a step in the right direction.[6,15,20,21]

ED APNs have another hurdle, specifically lack of standards of what is an acceptable educational background to work in the ED. There are few

schools with specific programs for emergency NPs, yet the number of NPs in the ED is growing every year. Because there is no standard for advanced nursing practice specific to the ED setting, there is no APN certification available to show that an NP has the minimum skills and knowledge necessary to practice in the ED. The CNS faces similar issues because there is no CNS certification specific to emergency nursing. CNSs are even more limited than NPs in their selection of examinations.

Although the number of APNs is growing each year, the numbers of nurses working in EDs in the advanced practice role are still small. There is no easy answer regarding advanced certification for APNs in the ED; however, as the debate continues, it is important that APNs take an active role in resolution of this debate. There are several ways an ED ANP can advocate for this specialty certification: (1) by becoming a member of Emergency Nurses Association, (2) by becoming actively engaged in the organization, and (3) by being informed.

Table 20-3

Ten Recommendations for Reform of Current Regulatory System for Health Care[6,18,19]

1. States should use standardized and understandable language for health professions regulation and its functions to clearly describe them for consumers, provider organizations, businesses, and professions.
2. States should standardize entry-to-practice requirements and limit them to competence assessments for health professions to facilitate the physical and professional mobility of health professions.
3. States should base practice acts on demonstrated initial and continuing competence. This process must allow and expect different professions to share overlapping scopes of practice. States should explore pathways to allow all professionals to provide services to the full extent of their current knowledge, training, experience, and skills.
4. States should redesign health professional boards and their functions to reflect the interdisciplinary and public accountability demands of the changing health care delivery system.
5. Boards should educate consumers to assist them in obtaining the information necessary to make decisions about practitioners and to improve the board's public accountability.
6. Boards should cooperate with other public and private organizations in collecting data on regulated health professions to support effective workforce planning.
7. States should require each board to develop, implement, and evaluate continuing competency requirements to ensure the continuing competence of regulated health care professionals.
8. States should maintain a fair, cost-effective and uniform disciplinary process to exclude incompetent practitioners to protect and promote the public's health.
9. States should develop evaluation tools that assess the objectives, successes, and shortcomings of their regulatory systems and bodies to best protect and promote the public's health.
10. States should understand the links, overlaps, and conflicts between their health care workforce regulatory systems and other systems that affect the education, regulation, and practice of health care practitioners and work to develop partnerships to streamline regulatory structures and processes.

Conclusion

Certification is a process that affects every APN because it is tied to the regulation of their practice. To date there is no certification to meet state regulation for licensure specific for APNs in the ED. The future of advanced practice is evolving. If certification is to become reality for the APN in emergency care, each and every APN currently working in an ED must work hard and diligently to make advanced certification a reality.

REFERENCES

1. Lewis, C., & Carson, W. (1998). Nurse practitioner certification: Benefits and drawbacks. *Advanced Practice Nursing Quarterly, 4*(3), 72–77.
2. McLeod, R. P. (1995). Nurse practitioners: Building on our past to meet future challenges. *Advanced Practice Nursing Quarterly, 1*(1), 15–20.
3. Porcher, F. K. (1999). Licensure, certification, and credentialing. In M. D. Mezey & D. O. McGivern (Eds.), *Nurse practitioners: Evolution to advanced practice* (pp. 422–433). New York: Springer.
4. National Council of State Boards of Nursing. (n.d.). *Nursing regulation.* Retrieved November 27, 2002 from http://www.ncsbn.org/public/regulation/licensure.htm
5. Mumma, C. (1998). Certification of advanced practice nurses. *Rehabilitation Nursing, 23*(3), 157–158.
6. Stanley, J. M., & Bednash, G. (1998). Formulation and approval of credentialing and clinical privileges. In C. M. Sheehy & M. C. McCarthy (Eds.), *Advanced practice nursing: Emphasizing common roles* (pp. 138–167). Philadelphia: F. A. Davis.
7. Fabrey, L. J. (1996). Basic psychometric principles. In A. H. Browning, A. C. Bugbee, Jr., & M. A. Mullins (Eds.), *Certification: A NOCA handbook* (pp. 1–40). Washington, DC: National Association for Competency Assurance.
8. Barkley, T. W., Haskin, R. C., & Tejedor, M. A. (2001). Practice issues: Credentialing, prescriptive authority, and liability. *Nurse Practitioner Forum, 12*(2), 106–114.
9. Buppert, C. (1999). What is a nurse practitioner? In C. Buppert (Ed.), *Nurse practitioner's business practice & legal guide* (pp. 1–39). Gaithersburg, MD: Aspen.
10. Felton, G. (1998). Politicization of health professions regulation. *Advanced Practice Nursing Quarterly, 4*(3), 14–23.
11. Buppert, C. (1999). State regulation of nurse practitioner practice. In C. Buppert (Ed.), *Nurse practitioner's business practice & legal guide* (pp. 104–124). Gaithersburg, MD: Aspen.
12. Romaine-Davis, A. (1997). Legal and licensing aspects of nursing. In A. Romaine-Davis (Ed.), *Advanced practice nurses* (pp. 23–35). Boston: Jones and Bartlett Publishers.

13. National Council of State Boards of Nursing. (1998). *Using nurse practitioner certification. Certification for state nursing regulation: A historical perspective.* Retrieved November 26, 2002 from http://www.ncsbn.org/public/regulation/licensure_aprn_practitioner.htm

14. National Council of State Boards of Nursing. (2002). *Regulation of advanced practice nursing: 2002 national council of state boards of nursing position paper.* Retrieved November 26, 2002 from http://www.ncsbn.org/public/regulation/res/APRN_Position_Paper2002.pdf

15. Griffith, P. B., & Logan P. (1999). Licensure, certification, and institutional credentialing. In P. Logan (Ed.), *The principles of practice for the acute care nurse practitioner* (pp. 31–38). Stamford, CT: Appleton & Lange.

16. Emergency Nurses Association. (n.d.). *ENA history.* Retrieved November 26, 2002 from http://www.ena.org/about/history/

17. National Council of State Boards of Nursing. (2002). *Proposed revision to the uniform advanced practice registered nurse licensure/authority to practice requirements.* Retrieved November 26, 2002 from http://www.ncsbn.org/public/regulation/res/Proposed_revision_to_the_Uniform_requirements_for_Delegate.pdf

18. Professional Examination Service. (1999). Evaluation by external consultants. *PES News: Methods for Evaluating and Auditing Credentialing Programs, 19*(1). [Electronic version]. Retrieved November 26, 2002 from http://www.proexam.org/newletter/1999a/ancc.htm

19. Pew Health Professions Commission. (1995). *Reforming health care workforce regulation: Policy considerations for the 21st century. Report of the taskforce on health care workforce regulation.* [Electronic version]. Retrieved November 26, 2002 from http://www.futurehealth.ucsf.edu/pdf_files/reforming.pdf

20. American Association of Colleges of Nursing. (1998). *Certification and regulation of advanced practice nurses.* Retrieved November 26, 2002 from http://www.aacn.nche.edu/Publications/positions/cerreg.htm

21. Barnum, B. S. (1997). Licensure, certification, and accreditation. *Online Journal of Issues in Nursing.* Retrieved November 26, 2002 from http://www.nursingworld.org/ojin/tpc4/tpc4_2.htm

BIBLIOGRAPHY

Niebuhr, B. S. (1993). Credentialing of critical care nurses. *AACN Clinical Issues in Critical Care Nursing, 4*(4), 611–616.

Pearson, L. (2002). Fourteenth annual legislative update. *The Nurse Practitioner: The American Journal of Primary Health Care, 27*(1), 10–12, 15, 19–20, 22–24, 26–30, 33–34, 37–40, 43–52.

21 | CREDENTIALING AND PRIVILEGING

Edwin W. Schaefer, ND, RN, FNP

After an advanced practice nurse (APN) has been offered and accepts a position, the credentialing and privileging process must be completed at their place of employment. In the past this process was reserved for institutional environments only. However, because of the increasingly litigious environment in health care, more private offices are requiring APNs to become credentialed and privileged within their practice setting. This process allows hiring institutions and groups to investigate the APN's professional credentials. The practice settings can then confirm credentials and certifications and decide if there are other issues that are pertinent to the APN and the ability to work in the organization (litigation, criminal offenses, etc.). Accrediting organizations query the National Practitioner Data Bank (NPDB) to determine if there are any proceedings pending or filed against the APN. This procedure needs to be repeated on a regular basis, usually every two years.[3]

History

The credentialing and privileging process was developed from requirements by the Joint Commission on Accreditation of Healthcare Organizations (JCAHO), Accreditation Association of Ambulatory Health Care, the National Committee for Quality Assurance, and the growing public awareness of the need for hospitals to protect the public health and safety. Credentialing and privileging also help organizations ensure that they provide quality care and avoid litigation. Initially the credentialing and privileging process was started for physicians only; however, now it involves other licensed professionals as well. The responsibility for credentialing and privileging rests with the highest level of the institution. This may be the board of directors or senior executive committee.

Their decision is based on information gathered during the credentialing process and from recommendations from the medical staff committees.[1,2]

The process for credentialing and privileging should be found in the medical staff bylaws, policies, and procedures. There should also be a process that allows for appeals. These manuals should be located in the institution's library, in the human resources department, or with the office manager.

Definitions

Licensure

Licensure is the legal permission to practice within a specific scope of practice once educational requirements have been met, a national examination has been successfully completed, and necessary fees have been submitted. Licensure indicates that the minimum requirements to practice at a certain level have been met. State government regulates this process through the state nurse practice act.[1]

Privileging

Privileging is the process that health care organizations use to determine the specific procedures and treatments that each health care practitioner may perform. The privileging list is a listing of procedures and conditions on which applicants check those they would like to be able to perform or treat (see Appendix A). The committee reviewing the privileging process examines the applicant's education and experience with each procedure and then grants permission to the practitioner to perform specific procedures or other patient care services. These privileges need to be

within the scope of practice for the individual, they need to be allowed by the individual's professional license, and the individual needs to have relevant training and experience to perform them.[1,2]

The privileging process typically has three aspects:

- Determining the clinical procedures and treatments that should be offered to the patients
- Determining the training and experience required to carry out each procedure or treatment
- Evaluating the qualifications of the applicant to approve or deny requested privileges

Credentialing

JCAHO defines credentialing as the process of assessing and validating the qualification of a licensed independent practitioner to provide patient care services in a hospital.[3] The determination is based on an evaluation of the individual's current license, training or experience, current competence, and ability to perform the privileges requested. The credentialing process is the basis for making appointments to the medical staff, and it also provides information for the process of granting clinical privileges to all licensed independent practitioners in the hospital.[3] It is important to note that the process the medical staff office completes to credential licensed independent practitioners is usually identical to the process that personnel and human resources departments use to verify the qualification of nurses and other allied health professionals seeking employment.

National Practitioner Data Bank (NPDB)

The NPDB is a national registry for physicians, dentists, nurse practitioners (NPs), and other health care professionals, which was established in 1989 by the federal government in response to the Health Care Quality Improvement Act of 1986. The NPDB tracks and reports incidents of poor or low-quality care of individual practitioners. It is primarily an alerting or flagging system intended to facilitate a comprehensive review of health care professionals' credentials. The NPDB acts as a

clearinghouse of information relating to the medical malpractice payments and adverse actions taken against the licenses, clinical privileges, and professional society memberships of physicians, dentists, NPs, and other health care professionals. Hospitals must report any negative professional review actions against health care professionals to the NPDB.[1] Examples of what must be reported are listed in Table 21-1.

Temporary Privileges

In certain circumstances, for example, when "important patient care needs mandate immediate authorization to practice," temporary privileges can be granted to new or existing medical staff or licensed professionals.[3] An example of an acceptable circumstance is if a physician becomes ill and takes a leave of absence, which requires coverage by another physician or licensed practitioner during the absence. Temporary privileges can be granted for a limited time up to 120 days by the chief executive officer with recommendation by the clinical department or president of the medical staff after verification of current licensure and competences and query of the NPDB.

Procedure

Each institution will have a slightly different procedure for credentialing and privileging, and the APN should become familiar with their specific institution's procedure. Usually an application will

Table 21-1
Items of Reportable Actions
<ul><li>Reduction in clinical privileges of greater than 30 days</li><li>Resignation</li><li>Surrender of privileges</li><li>Acceptance of privilege reduction either during investigation or to avoid investigation</li><li>Insurers must report any payments made for a licensed health care provider that results from a written claim or judgment. The law and JCAHO mandate that hospitals contact the NPDB for practitioners seeking initial appointments and thereafter every two years.[3] Because of this, most reappointments or recredentialing occur in two-year cycles.</li></ul>

be forwarded to the applicant indicating the type of references and supporting information that is needed to accompany the application. This process is laborious and can take up to six months to complete.[1]

Once the application is submitted, a human resources or medical staff person will call and confirm the references. The application will then be forwarded to a medical staff committee for consideration. The committee will review and decide if the information is sufficient for the position for which the person has applied. Usually physicians in the APN's practice or practice area will have discussed the application with the committee, and the approval should be uncomplicated. Table 21-2 includes information usually requested during the credentialing process.

The privileging mechanism needs to be hospital specific. APNs must seek and be granted privileges within each institution in which they intend to practice.[3] It is ultimately up to the individual institution to choose the best method of properly credentialing applicants that the hospital classifies as licensed independent practitioners (LIPs) or allied health professionals (AHPs). JCAHO states that LIPs should be credentialed through the same process as doctors, dentists, and podiatrists.[1] AHPs may be credentialed differently, for example, through the human resources department. Therefore it is important to determine how the institution defines APNs—either as LIPs or AHPs. NPs may fit either category, depending on the specific state rules and regulations. If the NP is considered an LIP, they will need to be credentialed by the hospital to be granted the privilege of performing medical acts within the institution. They may or may not hold a medical staff appointment.

Credentialing and privileging are required to legitimize the APN's practice and help to ensure professional accountability.[1] Because of this process, other organizations, such as government and private organizations, are more comfortable ensuring that APNs are providing safe care. This helps APNs be recognized as practitioners that are entitled to reimbursement. Many insurance companies or government programs require that providers meet a minimum standard before agreeing to reimburse for their care.

Table 21-2
Information Requested During the Credentialing Process
■ Copy of nursing license and APN license if applicable
■ Proof of education: transcripts, diploma
■ Copy of all certifications: NP, CPR, ACLS, PALS, ENPC, etc.
■ DEA number if applicable
■ Clinical references
■ Résumé/Curriculum vitae
■ Privileging form: This would be filled out by the APN and should include the specific privileges requested
■ Collaborative agreement (if applicable)

Economic Credentialing

It is important to provide high-quality care that is still efficient and cost effective. Some institutions and physician groups are beginning to look at ways to make practitioners more accountable for their care. One way to accomplish this is to look at cost factors or patient satisfaction scores to determine if the practitioner should be credentialed into the practice or be recredentialed. This type of economic credentialing would occur in addition to the current credentialing process.[4]

It is important for practitioners to know how they are being evaluated. This will be important to APNs for their evaluation of performance and their ability to be recredentialed in the future. Subsequent salary increases are usually attached to these measures.

Restraint of Trade

APNs that are not granted privileges because of unclear reasons can seek damages under restraint of trade. There can be political pressure brought to bear that restricts the ability of APNs to gain approval for their application. This could be related to economic or professional competition. There are legal remedies including restraint of trade, antitrust, and other forms of discrimination that can be pursued.[1,5] Using these options should be reserved for very specialized and extenuating circumstances and after all other avenues of resolution have been attempted, including appeals.

Becoming politically active and speaking to physicians and others that will be involved with the credentialing and privileging process would be wise. Having the APN's collaborating physician get a feel from the committee regarding the application can give the APN time to respond to concerns before they become issues that are difficult to resolve. APNs in the organization can be a valuable resource. Use them if that option is available.

Conclusion

Credentialing and privileging are important components of the medical staff office's responsibilities. The process began as a response to requirements set by several regulatory agencies. It is now an integral part of every health care institution, including hospitals, clinics, and office practices. Credentialing and privileging helps to ensure quality patient care. The APN must have a working knowledge of this process and submit required information in a timely manner during the application and recertification processes.

REFERENCES

1. Kamajian, M. F., Mitchell, S. A., & Fruth, R. A. (1999). Credentialing and privileging of advanced practice nurses. *AACN Clinical Issues, 10*(3), 316–336.
2. Hravnak, M., & Baldisseri, M. (1997). Credentialing and privileging: Insight into the process for acute-care nurse practitioners. *AACN Clinical Issues, 8*(1), 108–115.
3. Joint Commission on Accreditation of Healthcare Organizations. (2002). *Comprehensive accreditation manual for hospitals: The official handbook.* Oakbrook Terrace, IL: Author.
4. Baik, S. Y., Oakley, L. D., Hoebeke, R., & Dunham, N. C. (2001). Understanding managed care: Practice implications for NPs. *Clinical Excellence for Nurse Practitioners, 5*(4), 232–239.
5. Grad, J. D. (1982). Allied health professionals and hospital privileges: An introduction to the issues. *Law, Medicine and Health Care, 10*(4), 165–167.

Appendix A
GENERIC HOSPITAL

Emergency Nurse Practitioner
Privileging Form

Name: _____ Date: _____

Definition:

Collaboration: To communicate with a physician regarding treatment plan or procedure. The level of communication will be determined by patient acuity, treatment protocol, and/or the collaborative agreement. *(This definition will depend on the state in which you are practicing. This document should be reviewed by legal counsel familiar with advanced practice laws in the state in which it will be used.)*

Noncomplex: Determined by the presenting signs and symptoms and/or by a physician that examined or is consulted about the patient.

Return demonstration: To demonstrate and/or explain to a fully credentialed physician on staff the specific procedure or technique described.

Privileges			Privileges Granted	
Requested	Not Requested		Yes	No
		GENERAL		
		Complete a history and physical on patients presenting for care		
		Document all data on emergency department medical record		
		Order routine tests as deemed necessary by patient history, physical exam, and/or physician collaboration		
		Transcribe orders for medications/testing/ancillary services to medical record with MD cosignature		
		Order and administer medications as dictated by presenting signs and symptoms, treatment protocols, physician collaboration, and to the extent allowed by state laws		
		Assist in education of patients and their families and provide emotional support and referrals for financial, social, or other assistance		
		Consultation and referrals to physicians and various agencies and in scheduling of diagnostic and therapeutic procedures		
		Noncomplex care of patients presenting for treatment		
		Stabilization of patients requiring complex care		

		WOUND CARE		
		Order/administer topical anesthesia (ex: LET)		
		Local anesthesia infiltration		
		Administer regional blocks:		
		■ Digital block with successful return demonstration documented		
		■ Ankle block with successful return demonstration documented		
		■ Wrist block with successful return demonstration documented		
		Conscious sedation per protocol and physician collaboration		
		Noncomplex burn care (involving less then 10% TBSA)		
		Noncomplex wound care:		
		■ Noncomplex laceration repair with successful return demonstration of 10 varying repairs documented		
		Noncomplex foreign body removal		
		ORTHOPEDIC CARE		
		Reduction of noncomplex dislocations with collaboration of physician and successful return demonstration documented		
		Noncomplex fracture care:		
		■ Splint applications		
		■ Emergency mobilization technique and transportation		
		■ Closed reduction of noncomplex fractures		
		HEENT CARE		
		Noncomplex HEENT care		
		Anterior nasal packing/cautery		
		Use of slit lamp with successful return demonstration documented		
		Staining of eyes and Wood's lamp examination		
		Noncomplex foreign body removal		

		OTHER		
		Assessment and treatment of genitourinary complaints, including performing pelvic examinations with collections of cultures and Pap smears		
		Vascular access techniques (ex: IV access, ABG sampling, external jugular access, venous blood sampling)		
		Care of poisoning, drug overdose, and toxic ingestion		
		Gastric lavage		
		Urethral catheterization		
		Lumbar puncture with successful return demonstration documented		
		Mild to moderate conscious sedation following protocols and with physician collaboration		
		EMERGENT CARE		
		Initiate advanced cardiac life support treatment as dictated by patient need and/or protocol with physician collaboration		
		Initiate pediatric life support treatment as dictated by patient need and/or protocol with physician collaboration		
		Initiate trauma life support treatment as dictated by patient need and/or protocol with physician collaboration		
		Initiate and/or assist with precipitous delivery as dictated by patient need and/or protocol with physician collaboration		

_____   _____

Applicant   Date

_____   _____

Collaborating Physician   Date

_____   _____

Emergency Department Medical Director   Date

_____   _____

Chairman, Privileging Committee   Date

This is a sample Privileging List and may be reproduced. The author and/or Emergency Nurses Association have no responsibility or liability for any untoward actions resulting from the use of this form or any part of this form.

It is highly recommended that this form, if used, be reviewed by legal counsel familiar with advanced practice nursing law in the state the form will be used in.

22 WRITING FOR PUBLICATION: WHAT CAN ADVANCED PRACTICE NURSES WRITE ABOUT FOR PUBLICATION, AND HOW CAN THEY ENSURE THAT IT IS PUBLISHED?

Gail Pisarcik Lenehan, RN, EdD, FAAN

"I've Been an ANP for 10 Years, But I Really Don't Feel as Though I Am Expert Enough to Write for Publication."

This is a common sentiment, but advanced practice nurses (APNs), even those who don't think they have a thing to write about, are often the best source of journal articles. The job of a journal is to keep readers updated with the latest trends in a given field. If you are working in that field, you may have more to report than you think. Using the specialty of emergency nursing and one specialty nursing journal—the *Journal of Emergency Nursing**—as examples, let me illustrate this and other points.

Case Reviews

Start with the last interesting patient for which you cared. You are surely an expert on that patient. You know, more than anyone, what the patient's symptoms were, how you came to the diagnosis, what you did for that patient, how the patient responded to treatments and therapies, and what you learned. If you think that you did, in fact, learn from the case, and if you think what you learned was valuable information or insight for you—and that is a very key "if"—then readers may find teaching value in it as well. So

try a Case Review. Perhaps a recent patient with a tricyclic overdose who became obtunded and apneic within minutes taught you to make sure that such patients are always intubated early. Or perhaps you learned how strikingly a patient with Lyme disease mimicked a patient with multiple sclerosis and was almost sent out without beginning urgently necessary antibiotic therapy. Highlighting these patients through the vehicle of an actual case can be a powerful way to bring these teaching points home and keep readers up-to-date with current practice. If a patient's presentation and course taught you something, it may be valuable to pass on to others.

As an APN, you are in a position to see more cases of a certain type, to explore them in depth, and to grasp the big picture. A trauma nurse practitioner (NP) at a large regional trauma center, for example, recently reported a case of tracheobronchial injury. Her extensive experience, along with her knowledge of the most recent studies from the trauma literature, informed her rich discussion.[1]

Case Vignettes

You could also present several case vignettes to illustrate a point. A brief but powerful article published in the *Journal of Emergency Nursing* illustrates this technique. The article was written

**Journal of Emergency Nursing*

Gail Pisarcik Lenehan, RN, EdD, FAAN, Editor, P.O. Box 489, Downers Grove, IL 60515. Phone: 800-900-9659. FAX: 630-663-1273. E-mail link: glenehan@aol.com.

Managing Editor (for administrative/logistical questions): karen.halm@attbi.com

Author guidelines, tips for writing reports of research, intent to submit form, list of topics needed, submission deadlines: www.ena.org/publications/jen/index.htm

by an NP who reported on five patients that came to an emergency department (ED) with balanitis, an inflammation of the glans penis, within a year's period of time.[2] All five of them were found to be diabetic. The teaching point was to have a high index of suspicion for diabetes and send off urine and blood to check for glucose. After reading this article, other APNs may more readily think of sending off a blood sugar when they see a patient with balanitis or even another unexplained infection.

What Should I Write About?

Write about what you know. Few readers want to read the article written by an author who says, "Hhmm. 'Rape Trauma Syndrome' sounds interesting. I think I'll go to the library, look it up, and write something about that." Rather, readers want to hear from others who themselves have experience, research, or insights. Readers who work with children in severe pain from sickle cell crisis, for example, want to hear from someone such as an advanced practitioner at the Georgia Comprehensive Sickle Cell Center in Atlanta's Grady Health System about how to best treat their patients' pain.[3] For those who need to know how to set up an APN's emergency outpost in rural areas, readers might look to an APN who runs such a clinic in Northern Maine or Alaska. Who better to describe a new technique for digital block—the most common nerve block used in ED wound care—than a veteran ED NP who has used it in over 100 cases?[4]

One of my first articles was about patients who wanted to sign out "against medical advice."[5] It was a task gladly relegated to me as a psychiatric clinical nurse specialist (CNS) at Boston City Hospital's ED over the years, and I had become accomplished at helping such patients to stay and be treated. I knew a lot about the issue and had even delineated my own "typology" of such patients—those who were addicted and feared withdrawal if they were admitted, for instance, or patients in massive denial over their myocardial infarction (MI). In my advanced practice role, I had developed and tested various strategies that I had found helpful with each. The article described what worked and what didn't, which I

hoped would be helpful for staff in EDs that did not have someone in such a role. Another early article had to do with the role of the psychiatric CNS in the ED. My coauthors and I, working in the expanded role at Boston City's ED, had been encouraged to report the role in the literature for many months by our then ED Director of Nursing, Pam Maclean Johannsen, RN, MS, and we finally did it.[6]

An APN specializing in work with terminally ill patients in a hospice might want to write a practical article for emergency nurses about the latest interventions to treat pain and anxiety in dying patients or the myths that prevent them from being used. That same hospice APN might write another article, on the same topic, but this time for APNs, that would go into more depth about the aspects of what an APN would consider when prescribing such medications—contraindications, possible problems when combined with other medications, or how to use a combination of drugs for their synergistic effects, for example. Conversely, an ED NP might write an article for a hospice nursing journal about dealing with acute respiratory distress in a dying patient.

If you have implemented a program, perhaps one in which APNs are being used successfully and cost effectively in an ED, a hospice, or a shelter for the homeless, for example, share that information with others so that they can replicate your experience.

To What Journal Should I Submit My Manuscript?

Selecting which journal to submit your manuscript to is an important step in getting published. To find a list of nursing journals, consult the reference librarian of any library. There are also many guides to journals in nursing and related health fields. They list current journals, their preferred content areas, circulation, frequency, types of articles, whether they will publish student papers or revised theses, or whether they accept unsolicited manuscripts. There are also articles such as the classic, "Publishing Opportunities for Nurses: A Comparison of 92 U.S. Journals,"[7] which tell you such things as whether articles are

staff written, what percentage of articles are unsolicited, what the acceptance rate is, what percentage of articles are research, or how long it takes for acceptance and publication.

You can also search the Internet on these Web sites:

- ONLINE Nursing Editors, from the publication *Nurse Author and Editor* (http://www.members.aol.com/suzannehj/naed.htm), provides links to the Web sites of over 170 nursing journals and book publishers and gives direct e-mail links to their editors.
- The University of Texas, Medical Branch, School of Nursing Academic Journal Directory (http://www.son.utmb.edu/catalog/ajdindex.htm) lists journals in alphabetical order, by subject (such as emergency and critical care nursing journals), and by keyword search.

Here are some considerations when choosing a journal.

You can choose a journal by its audience. If you are an ED NP or an ED CNS with a depth of information on your specialty and have valuable information for other APNs or staff nurses in the ED, then choose the *Journal of Emergency Nursing.* You might also use your expertise to share information with a broader audience and publish in a more general nursing journal. For example, an ED NP might want to share an update with medical surgical nurses about the latest in resuscitation techniques, drugs, and defibrillation—what to do until the code team comes—or what the latest thinking is about the Trendelenburg position.

You can choose a journal by the fact of its credibility and prestige. In general, peer-reviewed journals hold more credibility. These journals have peers—reviewers with the same clinical or other expertise—review your manuscript, comment on its validity and worthiness, ask for revisions, and recommend acceptance or rejection. Journals that report a significant amount of research are also more prestigious. Journals that are "single-sponsor" publications, published by one drug company, for example, would be less prestigious.

You can choose a journal by its circulation. Some journals, such as the *American Journal of Nursing (AJN)* or *Nursing,* have circulations of over

300,000. *Nursing Spectrum,* a weekly nursing newspaper, has an aggregate 1 million readers across the country. Other journals, such as the official journal of a small nursing specialty group, may have only 2,000 subscribers. The *Journal of Emergency Nursing* has one of the largest circulations within the specialty nursing journals.

You can choose a journal that may help your career. If you want to move toward teaching or administration, it would bolster your résumé to publish in an educational or administrative journal. For example, manuscripts about a statewide continuing education program for emergency nurses or a successful ED nurse internship program for new graduate nurses would be welcomed in an educational or administrative journal as well as an emergency nursing journal.

Deciding where to send a manuscript is a matter of striking a balance between the journal in which you would like your manuscript to appear and the journal that will likely want your manuscript.

Make sure that the journal you choose is philosophically consistent with your topic. If you have a report of research or a review article that concludes that NPs are better able to assess or manage certain patients and do it less expensively than physicians, the staff of a physicians' journal might be more critical of your manuscript or feel that it was not a high priority for publication. Journals, particularly society-sponsored journals, have not just a readership but also a constituency and a mission, and they are important. This hypothetical manuscript might be more readily embraced, for example, by an APN journal, or a nursing journal with APN readers and a philosophy of support for nurses in advanced practice roles. But you want to get your message out to the nonbelievers, you say? Then consider a journal for nursing administrators or hospital administrators. Remember, your case will be stronger if you have compelling data or new information specifically targeted to the audience and if you talk the language of the average readers. To find the best journal in this instance, ask the administrators at your facility which journals they read.

Can't I Just Write the Article and Then Send It to a Number of Journals to See Which One Wants It?

No! All journals expect that manuscripts be submitted exclusively to them. To do otherwise would appear unethical. Here's why: When a manuscript is sent to a journal, that journal invests a great deal of time and energy in it. In peer-reviewed journals, the editor—often a volunteer—and three or more peers with expertise—often volunteers and often busy—read the manuscript carefully, sometimes multiple times, to make sure the information is valid and the style appropriate. They give thought to the manuscript, sometimes researching clinical information and checking references. They write down their impressions and suggestions for changes and deliberate over whether to recommend acceptance, revision, or rejection. With larger, more commercial journals, paid staff members may spend time working on the manuscript. After this investment, a journal would be very displeased to learn that the author had decided to place the article in a different journal.

The right thing to do is to send a manuscript to one journal at a time. Try to make sure that you get it back as quickly as possible from a journal so that you can send it elsewhere if it is rejected. It is the author's prerogative to inquire about whether a decision has been made after approximately six weeks and to encourage the editorial process along. A friendly informal note from the author to the editor asking about whether a decision has been made or whether the author can answer any questions or help with a review process is reasonable and appropriate.

The best way to make sure an article is accepted is to write it in the style, voice, and format of the articles already published in a particular journal. No journal temporarily suspends its normal style completely for one single manuscript, so look at the journal to which you are submitting. Make your manuscript "fit." Occasionally, journal editors receive a manuscript from an author saying something to the effect of, "Here is my manuscript. Feel free to edit it as you wish." Although a couple of the largest general-circulation journals have paid staff to work with manuscripts, most of the peer-reviewed specialty journals have no clinical editing staff or developmental editors. You are expected to revise as requested. You can save considerable time and energy by carefully reading one issue of the journal to which you are submitting. Look at an average article, and most importantly, look at the author guidelines. Specifically, verify the journal's page limit and the reference style.

Interestingly, in the revision request for the manuscript on the role of the psychiatric CNS that I mentioned earlier, the *AJN* associate editor asked us to cut the manuscript in half and add case examples. We could have anticipated these exact requests if we had simply read the author guidelines, which noted a page limit of 10 typed pages and encouraged the use of case examples. Our manuscript was 20 pages long and included no case examples. A careful look through the journal itself would also have yielded this information. At the time, the journal featured numerous case examples, and very few articles were longer than three journal pages (which is roughly equal to six to eight typed pages).

What Format Should I Use?

At the same time you are thinking about what to write and about where to publish, also give some thought to your format. Nursing journals offer more options than the journals of other specialties, which may feature only reports of research. There are case reviews, legal columns, "What's new?" columns, drug columns, or columns with questions and answers. Consider beginning with something as simple as a letter to the editor or a book review. If you know of a new book, video, or Web site that you found helpful, a nursing editor would probably welcome a review. For reporting research, the IMRAD (Introduction, Methods, Results, and Discussion) format is customary. For more in-depth suggestions on reporting research in this format, consult the *Journal of Emergency Nursing's* Web page at www.ena.org/publications/jen/index.htm

Because APNs are often breaking new ground at this time, we need descriptions of the successes and, even more important, failures that point out problems for which others should be aware.

Table 22-1

Reporting on Programs and Initiatives That You Have Tried in Your Facility	
Background/problem/situation before the program	■ What were the problems or needs, from the perspective of both patients and the institution that inspired the use of APNs?
Planning	■ How was the program planned? ■ Who was involved exactly? ■ How much time was spent in committee or individually to create the program? ■ What issues arose? ■ Were there turf issues? ■ What were the concerns or the resistance, and how were they dealt with? ■ What were the concerns raised? How were they resolved?
Program description	■ How, exactly, does it work? ■ For example, how is it staffed, what types of patients does the APN see, what is the cost, how is billing handled, what are the lines of reporting or responsibility, what is the structure for supervision?
Program evaluation	■ Did the program successfully address the original problem? ■ What else, if anything, did it accomplish? ■ What are the data to support its success or to show its lack of success (facts and figures)? ■ If no formal evaluation has been done, then what are typical comments from nurses, physicians, patients, and administrators?
Future plans for the program	■ Where do you see this program in 2, 5, or 10 years? ■ Will it stay the same, be expanded, or no longer be necessary after a few years?

Table 22-1 describes a sample format that can be used to report the use of APNs in an urban ED fast track or an Alaskan outpost clinic.

Any Pearls of Wisdom for the First-Time Author?

There are many books on writing and publishing for nurses, often in the reference section of nursing libraries. But none hold any lessons as valuable as the ones that you can easily learn from looking carefully at the journal in which you would like to publish. The 5 or 10 minutes that it takes to read a journal's author guidelines and skim the journal will save so much more time in the end. Take a careful look. What is the length of the articles? Each journal page is equal to about two and a half typed pages, double-spaced. Writing a longer piece means more work initially and then more work again when it has to be cut down. If most articles are three journal pages long, then assume that yours will be, too, sooner or later, one way or another. Get a sense of the style, the voice, and the various sections. Is the journal you are considering very practical and clinical? Even if

you would like to only write a letter, look at how long the letters generally are and the tone they assume.

The single most important thing to do before writing is to send a query letter or, even better, to call the editor. It saves time for the editor, as well as you, if you discuss the article early on, and most will welcome the letter, call, or even an e-mail note. When you call, be prepared to tell the editor your specific topic and its focus, what format you are thinking about using, what you will include in the article, and a little about why you are the best person to write about the topic. Ask if anything similar has been submitted, and gauge what the interest is. It is fine to be open and say that you are calling several journals to see which ones might be interested. If the editor is very enthusiastic, it will help motivate you to write.

Another strategy is to write something that you, yourself, would want to read. If you are writing for other APNs, and you find that what you are writing is exciting and interesting to read, rather than a chore to go over, then you are on the right

track. All too often, authors take a very interesting message and hide or bury it in passive, convoluted, stilted language. If you are writing for an audience other than APNs, ask someone from the intended audience to tell you the kinds of information within a topic that they most care about. Then make sure to address it. Staff nurses may say to include aspects of a clinical issue with which they are most concerned—how to best monitor a certain type of patient, perhaps, or ominous signs to be particularly aware of and alert the physician about. When you have something on paper, have someone from the intended audience review a draft and give you feedback.

It would also be helpful to develop a strategy for giving structure to your writing efforts. Create a schedule and write for the same two hours each day. Set aside a desk or table dedicated to writing, so you can pick up where you left off easily without losing your place. Give your manuscript some structure with subheads. If linear top to bottom outlining doesn't work, outline creatively. Put the main topic in the center and then jot down all of the aspects you would want to include around it. Then group subjects into subheadings. If you have initial blocks and can't decide how to begin a manuscript, jump into one of the subheadings that you are most comfortable writing about and begin there, in the middle. Ask yourself, "If I could include nothing else in this manuscript, what one thing would I most want to say to readers?" Write about that, and then ask the question, "If I could include nothing but two things in this manuscript. . . ."

Last but not least, remember that the perfect is often the enemy of the good. Convince yourself that your first words do not have to be profound. Tell yourself to write a "zero draft"—something that isn't at all polished or comprehensive, but is simply somewhere to begin. A good piece of writing is like a sculpture that you keep making better. But to sculpt, you have to have some clay. To fashion a manuscript, you have to begin with some words. You will make those words better and better, but you have to begin somewhere. Then step back, revise, move a paragraph from the end to the beginning, condense some material, or add some clarification, depth, or case vignettes.

What Are the Pitfalls to Avoid?

Avoid writing medical book chapters when writing for journals. Instead, write about what's new. The job of a journal is to keep its professional readers updated—to tell them what's new in the field, not to give basics that were covered in nursing school. ED APNs, for example, might write about what new drugs ED clinicians are using or drugs of abuse they see being abused on the street. You might describe trends such as overcrowding or increased workplace violence in EDs or a lack of in-service education in EDs and what is being done to address the problem.

Don't write about too broad a topic. You cannot write about "The Care of the Acute MI Patient" in, say, 10 pages. It will, of necessity, be superficial. There is just too much to cover. Instead, write with more depth, and focus your article. Write something such as "The Care of the Patient with an Acute MI: The First Five Minutes" or "Update on Thrombolytic Therapy for Patients with an Acute MI." You could also write an update about the latest technology—defibrillators or invasive monitoring devices used in the care of the acute MI patient. Consider sharing protocols, CareMaps®, guidelines, and flow sheets. APNs are often involved in writing these types of documents. Readers who adopt such a template from another facility can save themselves many hours of committee work. Just add a few words about anything that would not be apparent by just looking at the document. For example, have there been any problems or confusion with the guideline or form? What changes, if any, have been made since it was created, and why? What will be added or changed when it is next revised? How, exactly, is the tool used? How was the guideline in-serviced? What kind of in-service instruction about it has been used?

Avoid wordiness and jargon, the "optimize—maximize—utilize" syndrome. Would-be authors may mistake the use of jargon, polysyllabic, ostentatious words, and drawn out sentences for good writing. The truth? You can almost judge how good a piece of writing is by how short the words and sentences are.

Avoid vague, glowing generalities about how good or how important a program or clinical strategy is. Instead, give readers specifics and details. By the same token, don't tell readers what to do. Instead, tell them what, exactly, you did. Too many manuscripts say, "Nurses should . . ." or "Nurses must always. . . ." Instead, simply give readers the facts. Rather than saying that vital signs should be taken frequently on a certain type of patient, tell readers how quickly their blood pressure can drop, or how often the protocol at your institution requires that vitals be taken. This is a more compelling way to change practice.

If you are writing in a group, be aware that one person usually ends up making the writing of the various coauthors flow, coordinating with the group and the journal, obtaining permissions to use tables or illustrations, communicating with the journal, gathering additional information and permissions, and revising, sometimes more than once. It may be wise to determine who will be that one person and designate them as first author early on. This should not be done lightly, because more ownership is generally accorded to the first author.

How Can I Prevent Rejection?

The best insurance that your manuscript will be accepted is to have something compelling and worthwhile to say. The nursing literature is about improving the care of patients and the practice of nurses, and the articles that are truly valuable have the potential to change practice in some way.

If this is the case, then the next best strategy is to make your manuscript fit into a specific column or section in a specific journal. Every journal has pigeonholes in which to fit content. One way or another, each manuscript needs to fit. Write about a topic that is appropriate for a specific journal, and write it in the style, voice, and format of the articles in that journal.

What Can I Do If My Manuscript Is Rejected?

In the vast majority of cases, particularly with specialty nursing journals in which the authors are probably specialty nurses who are familiar with the audience, the journal requests a revision. The *Journal of Emergency Nursing,* for example, probably rejects outright less than 5% of submissions. This percentage is probably higher with more generalist nursing journals. But if your manuscript is rejected, it is acceptable and understandable to ask why. You can call or write to the editor. It is best to approach this with a friendly call to request feedback that may help you avoid rejection in the future. You can also ask where your manuscript might be more appropriately submitted. It has been our experience that, in the course of such conversations, the manuscript that the author could and should write often becomes apparent. Maybe a relatively dull overview article really should have been a case review recounting a fascinating patient for which the author provided care. If nothing else, it is a chance to familiarize yourself with the journal and to make yourself known as a potential resource. You may, for example, be a perfect reviewer for manuscripts on certain topics.

REFERENCES

1. Harrahill, M. (2002). Tracheobronchial injuries. *Journal of Emergency Nursing, 28*(3), 265–266.
2. DeVitis, M. G. (1982). Balanitis associated with hyperglycemia. *Journal of Emergency Nursing, 8*(4), 164–165.
3. Platt, A., Eckman, J. R., Beasley, J., & Miller, G. (2002). Treating sickle cell pain: An update from the Georgia Comprehensive Sickle Cell Center. *Journal of Emergency Nursing, 28*(4), 297–303.
4. Flarity-Reed, K. (2002). Methods of digital block. *Journal of Emergency Nursing, 28*(4), 351–354.
5. Lenehan, G. P. [Pisarcik]. (1978). Counseling the patient who wants to sign out AMA. *Journal of Emergency Nursing, 4*(3), 43–45.
6. Lenehan, G. P. [Pisarcik], Zigmund, D., Summerfield, R., Mian, P., Johansen, P., & Deveraux, P. (1979). Psychiatric nurses in the emergency department. *American Journal of Nursing, 79*(7), 1264–1266.
7. Swanson, E. A., McCloskey, J. C., & Bodensteiner, A. (1991). Publishing opportunities for nurses: A comparison of 92 U.S. journals. *Image: Journal of Nursing Scholarship, 23*(1), 33–38.

23

EVALUATING THE ROLE OF THE ADVANCED PRACTICE NURSE

Susan M. Bednar, RN, MSN, ANP

Performance evaluations are a vital tool for the advanced practice nurse (APN) and serve as a report card to administrators, delineating how well the APN has performed in the past and also giving direction for future goals. Evaluations can affect pay, job security, promotions, and even restructuring. Institutions that credential and privilege APNs to perform advanced practice procedures can use evaluations as a tool to evaluate and recommend continuation of these privileges in the future. The most effective evaluations reveal outcome data that have demonstrated the APN's worth in quantitative or qualitative measures and can even serve as road maps for the year ahead. The body of this chapter will present an overview of the who, what, when, and how of APN evaluation. It is intended to serve as a guide for the novice APN and an update for the experienced APN.

Who Evaluates the APN?

Because the APN is an autonomous, independent practitioner, determining who will evaluate the APN can be a challenge. It is important that the APN knows, up front, who will conduct the performance evaluation. Negotiating this point is essential prior to signing an employment contract. Usually, multiple people contribute to the APN evaluation including administrators, collaborating physicians, colleagues, staff nurses, and most importantly, patients. This multidisciplinary role of the APN can lead to difficult and often erroneous evaluations. Although some physicians may fail to recognize or value the teaching/counseling role of the APN, nursing supervisors may not appreciate the expanded medical management incorporated into the role,[1] and patient feedback may be limited to their level of satisfaction with the care they received while hospitalized. Therefore, it is important for the APN to know who will contribute to

the evaluation so the APN role can be structured accordingly. The APN may need to educate the evaluator about aspects of the role of which they are unaware and make a case for a multidisciplinary evaluation that would give the employer an appreciation for the role of the APN. Using a minimalist approach, the APN evaluation should include a self-evaluation, a peer evaluation, and an administrator evaluation.

What Will Be Evaluated?

Ideally, the APN should be evaluated on the components of the job description, including both process and outcomes evaluations. In other words, it is not enough to measure just how well the APN completed expectations of the role, but how well the process was implemented.[2]

The emergency department (ED) APN role includes the components of clinical expertise, leadership, educator, consultant, research, and outcomes management. APNs need to have a thorough understanding of the job description for the role into which they are hired. An example of a typical job description is provided in Table 23-1. Although the general components of the APN role include aspects of both traditional nurse practitioner (NP) and clinical nurse specialist (CNS) roles, there is much discussion in the literature today regarding merging the CNS and NP roles. Though there are variations in the role preparation (Table 23-2), the NP and the CNS do share similar scopes of practice.[3] It is important for the APN to know each of the components of the role that are stressed in their current employment and how these roles are going to be measured. For example, although both CNS and NP programs emphasize physical assessment, NP programs focus more training in the development

Table 23-1

Job Responsibilities of the CNS/NP	
CNS	NP

Clinical Practice
■ Provides a clinical expert perspective
■ Collaborates with multidisciplinary team
■ Develops plans of care for patient
■ Initiates patient care conferences
	Clinical Practice
	■ Assessment of health status
	■ Obtains health history
	■ Physical exam
	■ Preventative screen
	  □ Identify risk
	  □ Records changes

Consultation ■ Identifies problems/sets realistic goals ■ Develops policy/procedures for pt. care ■ Reviews and updates nursing procedures ■ Develops unit specific competencies	**Diagnosis** ■ Collaborates with MD ■ Differential diagnosis ■ Identifies needs
Education ■ Provides information to health care team ■ Assesses educational needs of patients/families ■ Identifies learning needs of patient caregivers ■ Participates in continuing education	**Treatment Plan** ■ Orders appropriate tests ■ Prescribes appropriate drugs ■ Plans for patient education

Research
■ Monitors quality improvement initiatives
■ Disseminates current research findings
■ Monitors performance improvement activities
■ Identifies areas for clinical study
	Implements Plan
	■ Based on priorities
	■ Based on knowledge
	■ Situation specific
	■ Interprets data
	  □ Accurate prescriptions
	  □ Patient education
	  □ Appropriate referrals

Professional Practice ■ Remains current in area of expertise ■ Attends workshops/seminars ■ Maintains specialty certification ■ Networking ■ Professional presentations/publishing	**Evaluation of Outcomes** ■ Documents outcomes ■ Reassess and modify
Leadership ■ Leads in development of goals ■ Demonstrates understanding of health care issues	**Patient Education** ■ For patient and families ■ Promote client self-care ■ Promote optimal health
Communication Goals	**Specific Job Competencies** ■ Professional practice ■ Research ■ Networking ■ Publication
	Communication Goals

Used with permission: Evanston Northwestern Healthcare. (2002, May). *Job Description and Performance Appraisal.* (Form 27003, 27004). Evanston, IL: Author.

of diagnostic reasoning skills and clinical applications.[3] Therefore, the NP would want to be sure these components were measured in an evaluation.

To support and justify the APN role, the evaluation tool must address measurable outcomes.

Wojner describes outcomes management by the APN as optimizing outcomes through the provision of care guided by research and argues that APN education positions these nurses in a leadership role because of their specialized clinical ex-

Table 23-2		
Contrasting CNS and NP Curricula for APN Preparation		
SKILLS	CNS CURRICULUM	NP CURRICULUM
Physical assessment	Often limited to particular system	Comprehensive
Diagnostic reasoning	Limited	Curricular thread
Management of health problems	Limited; requiring approval of others	Comprehensive
Systems focus	Usually strong; addresses consultation	Often focused on individual; limited focus on context
Leadership	Strong focus	Variable
Interdisciplinary approach	Nurse to nurse	Nurse to physician
Autonomy	Limited	Essential; contributes to role crisis

Reprinted with permission from Gilliss, C. (2000). In J. Hickey, R. Ouimette, & S. Venegoni (Eds.), *Advanced practice nursing: Changing roles and clinical applications* (p. 39). Baltimore: Lippincott Williams & Wilkins.

pertise, research skills, and mastery of the change process.[4] In an era in which effectiveness is largely measured in financial outcomes and APNs find themselves in a position in which they are not generating revenue, outcomes management is of paramount importance in demonstrating their effectiveness.[5] Specific examples of outcomes should be included on the evaluation tool. An example of this is APN participation in the development of care paths/critical care paths, which can shorten a patient's length of stay. Membership on hospital committees, such as the products committee that reviews products used within the institution, is another way that the APN adds to cost containment. The numerous tasks that go into preparing for a Joint Commission on Accreditation of Healthcare Organizations survey and keeping the hospital in good standing should be noted on the APN evaluation. Table 23-3 outlines outcome measures used in APN effectiveness research.

APNs whose primary responsibility is in the care of ED patients need to demonstrate competence in treating patients along with timely follow-up and concise documentation. Using a competency profile can assist APNs in documenting expertise, situations, and priorities of their role over the preceding year.[1] All core APN skills should be addressed in the competency profile with explanations of how and when the competencies were met and updated. Incorporating education and

preventive strategies should also be a part of the care rendered and should be evaluated.[4]

Consultation is another role of the APN and may be conducted directly with the physicians in the ED or other staff or other professionals within the hospital, community, or health care arena. Consultation and consultative services must also be documented so they can be included in the overall evaluation of the APN.

A master's-prepared nurse is constantly involved in reading research and incorporating research into practice as an ongoing activity. The degree to which the APN is involved in research, whether it is in relaying current clinical findings, becoming a part of a research project, or heading up a research team, should be documented and evaluated annually.

In terms of outcomes, consider the ED population to be a small business, and keep track of the patients seen and care rendered from Day One. This allows the APN to demonstrate value on a daily basis and to pick up on health care trends and future directions.[5] For example, in this author's busy ED, the APNs tabulated the amount of time that each ED patient spent in fast track. Over a period of six months, the APNs noted an increase in wait times. After a thorough review of the situation, the APNs suggested that the main reason for the long turnaround times was a shortage of ED beds. Once this data was presented to administration,

Table 23-3

Outcome Measures Used in APN Effectiveness Research

CARE RELATED	PATIENT RELATED	PERFORMANCE RELATED
■ Cost ■ Length of stay ■ In-hospital mortality ■ Morbidity ■ Readmission rates ■ Occurrence of drug reactions ■ Procedure success rate/ complications ■ Clinic wait time ■ Time spent with patients ■ Number of visits per patient ■ Number of hospitalizations ■ Use/ordering of lab tests ■ Rate of drug prescription ■ Management of common medical problems ■ Number of consultations ■ Infant immunizations ■ Diagnoses made ■ Diagnostic screening tests ordered ■ Acute care home visits ■ Intravenous fluid volume ■ Total parenteral nutrition use ■ Number of blood transfusions ■ Prenatal/postpartum visits ■ Low birth weight rates ■ Rates of cesarean section ■ Number of induced labors ■ Use of fetal monitoring ■ Analgesia/anesthesia used ■ Forceps deliveries ■ Amniotomies ■ Apgar scores ■ Infant growth and development	■ Patient satisfaction ■ Patient access to care ■ Patient compliance ■ Patient complaints ■ Health maintenance ■ Return to work ■ Stress levels ■ Knowledge ■ Blood pressure control ■ Diet and weight control ■ Blood glucose levels ■ Clinic wait time ■ Emergency room wait time ■ Drug interactions ■ Alcohol consumption	■ Quality of care ■ Interpersonal skills ■ Technical quality ■ Completeness of documentation ■ Time spent in role components ■ NP job satisfaction ■ Clinical competence ■ Performance ratings ■ Collaboration ■ Procedure complication rates ■ Revenue generation ■ Physician recruitment and retention ■ Time savings for house staff MDs ■ Effect on MD workload ■ Adherence to best-practices guidelines ■ Index scores on management of common medical problems

Adapted from Kleinpell, R. (2001). *Outcome assessment in advanced practice nursing* (p. 5). New York: Springer.

ED bed capacity was expanded, and ED wait times once again decreased. The APN used this information to support and document a positive self-performance evaluation. When deciding what type of data to monitor, it is much easier to track prospective data than to have to go back and retrieve often-unattainable data. With this in mind, the APN needs to determine prospectively what evaluation data will be important to track for the upcoming year. Some common outcome measures for NPs are patient satisfaction scores, length of stay, emergency room wait time, and revenue generated (Table 23-3).

Whitcomb, Craig, and Welker[6] described a tool for outcomes evaluation for the APN in terms of using a monthly report tracking four major components: (1) APN interventions, (2) education, (3) committee involvement, and (4) professional activities. Each component has a set of evaluation criteria. The APN intervention component tracks specific patient care rendered and procedures completed for each patient (including history and physicals, orders, workups, and discharge). Education evaluation includes patient care conferences, educational presentations, certifications and updates, and competency validation. Other areas

tracked are projects, indirect care, patient visits, and consultations. By tracking theses activities monthly, the APN can better evaluate the role and clearly demonstrate value to the institution.

When Should the Evaluation Take Place?

Although most evaluations occur annually, it may behoove the new APN or an experienced APN who has moved into a new role to ask for a six-month evaluation just to be sure they are on track with the role expectations. Although yearly evaluations are the norm, it is wise for the APN to set goals at 3, 5, and 10 years and perform a self-evaluation yearly to see how these goals are being met. For example, an APN may wish to have a certain number of publications by year 3 or begin a research project by year 5.

How Will the APN Be Evaluated?

There are several methods available for APN evaluation. Following is a list of the most frequently used evaluations methods.

1. Self-evaluation
2. Annual report
3. Monthly reports
4. Peer review

Self-evaluation is one form of assessment for the APN to consider. Self-evaluation is an important function of a professional and should be utilized, even if it is not a requirement of the specific employer.[2,8,9] In self-evaluation, individuals rate themselves in regard to established performance criteria and their own personal goals. The process of self-evaluation gives APNs an opportunity to critically review their own performance and to develop goals for the future based on that evaluation.[9]

For some, an annual report that describes the activities and accomplishments of the previous year is used as the formal evaluation and the APN's self-evaluation.[8,9] If this is the case, then the job description and performance criteria can serve as a guide in preparing the report. The APN is encouraged to delineate each responsibility listed under the job description and document how this responsibility has been met. Additionally, the APN might find that doing ongoing monthly reports actually helps to keep documentation current and makes the final year-end report much easier.

Finally, peer review is a commonly used evaluation method. Peer review is the process by which people of the same rank, profession, and setting critically appraise each other's work. Some of the benefits of peer review are that it can increase professionalism, accountability, and teamwork among peers.[10,11] Peer review is best used as a self-development tool, and if done correctly, it can increase the cohesiveness of the group and can improve the quality of care provided as a whole.[10,11]

Quite simply, the tool that is used for evaluation needs to accurately reflect the APN's specific role, preferably, what the APN does on a daily basis. The evaluation form should reflect the components of the APN roles of expert clinician, leader, educator, consultant, researcher, and outcomes manager. Individual performance evaluations should also show compliance with federal, state, and institutional practice requirements (i.e., licensure, collaborative practice agreements). There should be a place to document goals met (along with dates) from the previous year and goals for the upcoming year, including target dates for completion of each component. Also, job-specific competencies should be included. This is paramount if the APNs need documentation to keep their privileges within an institution. For example, if the APN is to function in an urgent care setting, then some of the job competencies evaluated would include such tasks as suturing, accurate x-ray interpretation, and postmold applications. Figure 23-1 is an example of an evaluation tool used for APN providers in the ED at an urban/suburban Midwest hospital. This tool was designed through consultation with other colleagues from various institutions, who generously shared their useful evaluation tools and their experiences. The evaluation was then analyzed for a fit within the institution and was approved by both the APNs and the administration.

Two role expectations that merit special discussion are communication and professional development. Exceptional communication skills are an

FIGURE 23-1 *NP/PA Evaluation Form*

Nurse Practitioner/Physicians' Assistant Name:

Evaluator (Optional):

Date:

Please rate from 1–10 the following characteristics:

	[1–3 Superior]	[4–6 Satisfactory]	[7–10 Unsatisfactory]
I. Clinical Judgment/Clinical Skills			
1. Obtains a thorough and accurate health history	1 2 3	4 5 6	7 8 9 10
2. Performs comprehensive physical assessments and discriminates between normal and abnormal findings	1 2 3	4 5 6	7 8 9 10
3. Prioritizes health care needs and coordinates patient care in collaboration with physicians	1 2 3	4 5 6	7 8 9 10
4. Oral case presentations are clear, organized, and concise	1 2 3	4 5 6	7 8 9 10
5. Appropriate and complete organization of data in chart	1 2 3	4 5 6	7 8 9 10
II. Documentation	1 2 3	4 5 6	7 8 9 10
III. Patient Relations/Staff Relations			
1. Instructs and updates patients and families on therapeutic regimen	1 2 3	4 5 6	7 8 9 10
2. Able to relate effectively to patients and their families	1 2 3	4 5 6	7 8 9 10
3. Consults with other health care professionals as appropriate	1 2 3	4 5 6	7 8 9 10
4. Shares team responsibilities in providing care and follow-up for patients	1 2 3	4 5 6	7 8 9 10
5. Works well with members of the health care team	1 2 3	4 5 6	7 8 9 10
IV. Fund of Knowledge:			
1. Fund of Knowledge Appropriate fund of knowledge and understanding of disease processes	1 2 3	4 5 6	7 8 9 10
2. Problem Solving and Clinical Applications Appropriately integrates data, identifies clinical problems, and develops a plan of care	1 2 3	4 5 6	7 8 9 10
Specifies diagnostic strategies and treatment interventions	1 2 3	4 5 6	7 8 9 10
Evaluates patient responses to interventions and revises plan of care	1 2 3	4 5 6	7 8 9 10
V. Professional and Personal Attributes:			
1. Functions in a self-directed, autonomous manner, seeking input/ guidance when appropriate	1 2 3	4 5 6	7 8 9 10
2. Promotes clinical competence and the delivery of quality patient care	1 2 3	4 5 6	7 8 9 10
3. Maintains and updates clinical knowledge base and skills based on current health care practice, seminar attendance, and professional association membership	1 2 3	4 5 6	7 8 9 10

Room for Growth:

Overall Comments:

Emergency Department Nurse Practitioner Manual
Revision Date: October 23, 2001
Evanston Northwestern Hospital

expectation for all APNs and are integral components of the role. Part of the evaluation should reflect how well the APN communicates with other members of the health care team, patients, and families. APNs who communicate effectively are most likely to a have strong sense of their professional self.[12]

Professional development should also be demonstrated on the evaluations. The APN should set yearly goals for ongoing professional development, such as membership in a state, regional, or national organization (i.e., Emergency Nurses Association); educational development; certifications; publications; presentations; community involvement; or research activities. Professional development goals should be delineated as yearly, three-year, or five-year goals and be evaluated each year for progress.

According to Chinn,[13] being able to care and connect with others in a meaningful way depends fundamentally on one's own self-image and on the ability to care for one's self. In other words, "you cannot give that which you do not have." One strategy to help feed the well and fill the void is to find a mentor. The concept of mentoring is an essential component in the ability of APNs to actualize a positive future and can help the novice APN navigate through the constantly changing health care landscape. A strong mentor can guide the APN in practice and help pave the way for a successful evaluation for the novice APN.

Summary

APNs are true pioneers in the rapidly changing health care environment, and although this change brings opportunity, it also challenges APNs to reject the dependent stereotypes of the past. As APNs change from a dependent role to an independent role, the task of APNs is to prove their value. A major part of the APNs' role is to accept accountability and evaluate their effectiveness. This charge gives APNs cause to pause and reflect on their self-perception and the impact they make on the health care of the nation. Hickey[14] eloquently describes what might lie ahead for APNs:

As we contemplate the impact of healthcare changes on advanced practice nursing, the complexities and interrelatedness of the multiple systems and contextual layers that form the fiber of healthcare delivery are both immobilizing and empowering. Nurses cannot sit passively and let healthcare reform and the redesign of practice occur without a strong, active, and collective voice in shaping our own destiny. These are times of unprecedented opportunities for nursing; they are also times of risk and perils, for nothing is certain. . . . APNs must exercise their growing power to deliberately choose and create their collective futures so they can participate in meeting the healthcare needs of a nation.

It is through effective evaluations that APNs can prove their worth to society and their value within the health care arena. Through diligent attention to evaluation, APNs can demonstrate in measurable terms their unique contribution to the health care community. Specific job responsibilities for the APN were identified and described. Special mention was made on the importance of outcomes research in evaluation and specific role competencies. It was argued that along with outcomes data, a strong, positive professional self-concept is essential for the APN role to grow and flourish. The following advice from Dr. Seuss reminds us that with regard to APNs, the future is certainly what we make of it:[15]

> Congratulations!
> Today is your day
> You're off to great places
> You're off and away
> And oh, the places you'll go!!

REFERENCES

1. Brykczynski, K. A. (2000). Role development of the advanced practice nurse. In A. B. Hamric, J. A. Spross, & C. Hanson (Eds.), *Advanced nursing practice: An integrative approach* (2nd ed., pp. 107–134). Philadelphia: Saunders.
2. Hamric, A. (1989). A model for CNS evaluation. In A. B. Hamric & J. A. Spross (Eds.), *The clinical nurse specialist in theory and practice* (2nd ed., p. 101). Philadelphia: Saunders.
3. Gilliss, C. (2000). Education for advanced practice nursing. In J. Hickey, R. Ouimette, & S. Venegoni (Eds.), *Advanced practice nursing: Changing roles and clinical applications* (2nd ed., pp. 38–40). Baltimore: Lippincott Williams & Wilkins.

4. Wojner, A. (2000). Pushing the boundaries of advanced practice nursing. In J. Hickey, R. Ouimette, & S. Venegoni (Eds.), *Advanced practice nursing: Changing roles and clinical applications* (2nd ed., p. 462). Baltimore: Lippincott Williams & Wilkins.

5. Burns, S. (2001). Selecting advanced practice outcome measures. In R. Kleinpell (Ed.), *Outcome assessment in advanced practice nursing* (p. 73). New York: Springer.

6. Whitcomb, R., Craig, R., & Welker, C. (2000). Measure how ACNPs impact outcomes. *Nursing Management, 31*(3), 49–50.

7. Hawkins, J., & Thibodeau, J. A. (1993). *The advanced practitioner, current practice issues* (3rd ed.). New York: Tiresias Press.

8. Tye, C. C. (1997). The emergency nurse practitioner role in major accident and emergency departments: Professional issues and the research agenda. *Journal of Advanced Nursing, 26*(2), 364–370.

9. Ingersoll, G. L. (1995). Evaluation of the advanced practice nurse role in acute and specialty care. *Critical Care Nursing Clinics of North America, 7*(1), 25–33.

10. Winch, A. (1989). Peer support and peer review. In A. B. Hamric & J. A. Spross (Eds.), *The clinical nurse specialist in theory and practice* (2nd ed., pp. 251–256). Philadelphia: Saunders.

11. Blanton, N. E., Bogner, M. J., Collins, H. L., Futrell, J. A., Lagina, S., & Rolison, A. (1985). Putting peer review into practice. *American Nurse, 85*(11), 1284, 1287.

12. Courtney, R., & Rice, C. (1997). Investigation of nurse practitioner-patient interactions: Using the nurse practitioner rating form. *Nurse Practitioner, 22*(2), 46–48, 54–57, 60.

13. Chinn, P. (1991). Looking into the crystal ball: Positioning ourselves for the year 2000. *Nursing Outlook, 39*(6), 251–256.

14. Hickey, J. (2000). Advanced practice nursing in the dawn of the 21st century. In J. Hickey, R. Ouimette, & S. Venegoni (Eds.), *Advanced practice nursing: Changing roles and clinical applications* (2nd ed.). Baltimore: Lippincott Williams & Wilkins.

15. Seuss, Dr. (1990). *Oh, the places you'll go.* New York: Random House.

24

PUBLIC SPEAKING

Barbara A. Weintraub, RN, MSN, MPH, PCCNP, CEN

Oliver Wendell Holmes once said, "It is the province of knowledge to speak and it is the privilege of wisdom to listen."[1] As advanced practice nurses (APNs), we speak not only to educate on our topics themselves, but also on the role we play in the health care arena. It is through public speaking that we lend a face to our profession and legitimacy to our roles.

Communication skills for nurses are essential for numerous reasons. As nurses, we are charged with the collection, analysis, and dissemination of pertinent data. As APNs, we are expected to present our history and physical exam findings in a succinct, accurate manner. When there is a difference of opinion regarding a patient, we speak to influence opinion. Our colleagues, both physicians and nurses alike, expect us to present our analysis of a patient's case, a summary of a particular pathophysiology, or an explanation of a new medication or skill with grace and composure. Patients and their families demand explanations that are precise, to the point, compassionate, and imparted in layman's terms. All of these situations revolve around the ability to analyze, synthesize, and impart knowledge in various public forums. They are all aspects of professional speaking.

Although you may feel that public speaking is not your forte, consider that the need for oral communication skills is so high that the typical American gives approximately one dozen speeches per year in the course of employment. These speeches come in the form of staff meetings, parent-teacher conferences, patient rounds, in-services, and care conferences.[2]

Numerous articles from the 1980s and 1990s speak of the importance of public-speaking skills as a tool to "set us apart from the crowd."[3,4,5] One report indicated that oral communication was one of the seven "basic work place skills" wanted by employers,[2] and that communication skills rated second only to job knowledge as a factor in employee success, as well as being the primary indicator of a manager's success.[2] Research also indicates an increase in job satisfaction when we perceive our personal communication skills as high.[6,7]

For nurses to achieve professional autonomy, influence health care, and gain respect, we must learn to communicate who we are and what we do. One component of this strategy is making our voices heard in the public-speaking domain. As APNs, it is our professional duty to actively seek out opportunities to educate the public on who we are, what we know, and what we do.

Choice of Speaking Engagement

Public speaking consistently ranks high in surveys of most-feared situations. In some studies, it ranks higher than flying, financial difficulties, losing one's job, and death.[8] Therefore, an established strategy in preparation for speaking engagements is a key factor for a successful experience. There are two avenues to the public-speaking engagement. As an APN with a recognized area of expertise, you may be asked to speak on a given topic for which you are well known. However, we need not wait for offers to knock at the front door. An active quest for speaking engagements is a sensible option for those wishing to begin a public-speaking career.

If you are interested in becoming a public speaker and the opportunity has not yet presented itself, you should develop a strategy toward that end, treating the endeavor as a business venture. One experienced public speaker recommends first asking yourself, "What am I good at, and who needs

my skills?"[9] There are two basic markets for public speakers. The first is as an independent provider; this is usually more successful once you are an established, experienced speaker. The other option is to contract with a commercial company, a school, or a professional organization to speak on a specific topic. Regardless of which route you opt to follow, you will need an up-to-date curriculum vitae and references that speak to your experience as related to your topic.

When an opportunity for a public-speaking engagement presents itself, several factors must be evaluated before agreeing to accept the speaking commitment. It is vital to ensure that you are certain of what is expected of you prior to accepting a speaking engagement. The first factor to consider is the date of the engagement. Not only must the date be one for which you are available, but it must also be sufficiently far in the future to allow you adequate preparation time. Regardless of how eager you are to speak to a particular group or on a certain subject, there is no factor more certain to confound your ability to speak than having inadequate preparation time. One source cited an average preparation time of 100 hours for a one-hour presentation.[10]

Choice of topic is another key factor. The best results occur when the topic is one about which you are both knowledgeable and passionate. Although you may elect to speak on topics with which you are willing to become familiar, you will feel most confident when the topic is within your area of expertise.

When considering a speaking engagement, you should also inquire about the specific purpose of the speech, the demographics of the audience,[11] and the intended length of the presentation. Novice speakers may feel comfortable with a 30-minute presentation, but not with a one-hour presentation. Needless to say, the longer the presentation, the longer the preparation time required. This also requires a realistic look at other commitments that could interfere with adequate preparation time.

Knowledge of audience demographics is an essential component of successful professional presentations. Recognition of the needs of the audience is equally as important as choice of topic. An audience of school nurses expects to hear a different speech than does the PTA, and a mixed group of physicians, nurses, and allied health personnel should have an oratory that caters to their needs and knowledge levels as well. A careful assessment of the intended audience will allow you to fine-tune both the explicit and the latent messages within your speech to fit the needs characteristics of your intended audience.[11] In addition, a careful self-evaluation of your capacity to speak to the required group will ensure that you do not accept an engagement to speak to a group in front of whom you will not feel comfortable. A public speaker should also know the estimated size of the audience. This will help determine the type of audiovisuals selected, as well as the style of the presentation (e.g., a question-and-answer format would not be practical for a very large group).

Boundaries, scope, and depth will also revolve around the selected audience. The boundaries of a speech reflect the generality or specificity of your presentation. A presentation with wide boundaries reflects more of an overview of a topic, such as a speech on women's health, whereas narrow boundaries typically look at a very specific topic, such as the role of hormone replacement therapy in the postmenopausal woman. Boundaries may also reflect topics about which you should avoid speaking to certain groups, such as use of the morning after pill when speaking to an antiabortion group. Scope narrows the topic further (e.g., examination of the role of hormone replacement therapy in the prevention of osteoporosis in women over 65). Depth refers to the amount of detail covered in a presentation. For instance, the depth of a presentation to a group of nuclear physicists could go down to the atomic level.

As a professional, you should expect to receive an honorarium or fee for speaking. The amount you cite as your fee depends on numerous factors, including the type of organization for whom you are speaking (charitable versus profit driven), the type of speech (keynote versus one of a series of lecturers), the amount of preparation time required, and the size of the audience. If no specific fee is mentioned, do not hesitate to mention what your customary fee is, and let the discussion progress from there. Another factor to consider and discuss is coverage of any other related fees,

such as travel, accommodations, meals, or copying. Although as nurses we tend to think of payment in terms of altruism or lack thereof, in truth, our demeanor and demands, including payment of fees, contribute to the view that others hold of us. We want to be seen as the highly valued professionals that we are, so must we conduct our business transactions accordingly.

Once all of these components are established, you must determine whether or not you will accept the offer to speak. Many experienced speakers recommend against giving an immediate decision.[10,12] This gives you time to objectively assess your interest, experience, and capability against those required for the engagement. This is also the time to realistically assess your ability to meet the program deadlines, given your other commitments. If you elect to defer, thank the offering party for their invitation while respectfully declining the opportunity at this time. You should not delay your decision more than one to two weeks to allow the offering party time to find another speaker. If you decide to accept the offer, the time to begin preparation is at hand.

Speech Preparation

As previously discussed, speech preparation is time consuming. Proper planning and organization of a speech are essential to the success of a presentation.[11] A speech should be both well researched as well as supported by the literature. Begin with an analysis of your topic's central message.[12] What are the essential elements for the audience to take home? Are you seeking to persuade or inform? Setting realistic objectives at the outset will guide your outline first and then your presentation itself.

Regardless of your familiarity with a topic, a review of the literature should be the next step. Although you may not use all of the information you find, you will be better prepared, more confident, and more at ease with questions after a thorough review of the literature. Explore your topic in depth, utilizing a thorough computer search of nursing literature, as well as related disciplines. Speak to experts in the field to be directed to the latest research. Although you need not cite each source in your speech, each source

should be carefully documented. This is important for a number of reasons. If there is a question as to credibility, you will have the citations ready and at hand. In addition, questions may arise from the audience regarding study technique or seeking further information on a topic. A speaker gains both legitimacy and respect by having references at hand to disseminate. It is also to the speaker's advantage if the presentation is an overwhelming success, and he or she wishes to publish the speech as an article; the literature search and references are already completed.

Having now gathered all pertinent research and references, it is time to assemble the speech. Keep in mind that our purpose when speaking is to direct the minds of our listeners "along the narrow path of our own thoughts."[13] To do this requires us to verbally paint a picture through which we will lead our listeners. Proper organization of a speech will help hold the audience's interest and will establish you as the tour guide through the picture you hope to paint.

Although experienced speakers have all developed their own personal methodology to coordinating a professional presentation, they all share one key factor—organization. Communication is not the transmission of information, nor the mere speaking of facts and data, but rather the sharing of meaning.[2] Each presentation should be tailored to that specific audience at that specific time. Some presentations are best organized chronologically, some from most important to least important, or from least compelling to most compelling. Decide which method is correct for this particular presentation. Because an oral presentation is different from a written one, its preparation is different as well. Unless you are a very experienced presenter, the most effective method of preparation involves writing an overview of what you will say and then converting to the format from which you choose to speak.

A standard speech consists of an introduction, a body, and a conclusion. Many speakers paraphrase this as "tell them what you're going to tell them, tell them, then tell them what you told them."[14] One method to assembling your thoughts at this point is to take out four sheets of paper. On the top of the first, write "Introduction," on

sheet two write "Body," and on sheet three write "Conclusion." Sheet four is your "Other/Miscellaneous" sheet. Starting with the body of the speech, write down the three main points you wish to make on sheet two. Although there may be numerous relevant points, most polished speakers recommend keeping the main points to three[2,13] to keep the audience from getting lost in too many details.

Begin to flesh out each point with details to support your contentions. Again, limit the supporting evidence to no more than three points per detail. Supporting details can be facts, stories, or relevant research. Remember that the type of details you choose will help dictate the type of audiovisuals that you will use to make your point. Because the size of the audience also affects the type of audiovisuals used, the same presentation given to 10 people may end up with different supporting details than when given to 200 people. To help hold an audience's attention, one speaker recommends adding a story or anecdote every 15 to 20 minutes.[15]

Next, outline your introduction on the first page. Depending on the situation in which you are speaking, someone else may introduce you with your credentials, or you may be called on to introduce yourself. If someone else is not introducing you, it is important for you to introduce yourself to establish both credibility as well as some degree of familiarity.

There are many different schools of thought on what entails an effective opening remark. Although some recommend steering clear of humor, others feel that as long as the humor is not derogatory, that you are comfortable in relaying the humor, and that you know the audience is of the type to appreciate humor, it is an acceptable choice. Other successful opening remarks are relevant quotes, a purpose statement, or a startling statistic. The idea is to capture the audience's attention while giving them a brief glimpse of what is to come.

After you have completed the body of the speech and your introduction, you can begin to prepare your conclusion on page three. A conclusion has several purposes. Your conclusion should summarize the main points of your presentation. It should leave the audience invigorated, and wanting more. In addition, a conclusion should take advantage of the "primacy–recency" effect[2]—people are more likely to remember what they heard at the beginning and at the end of a presentation, rather than in the middle. Thus, the conclusion should be a powerful summation of what you would like each person to walk away with.

As you continue to flesh out the details of your speech, jot down points that you know you want to make in your speech but haven't placed yet in it on sheet four. This is also the place to write down ideas for audiovisuals that you want to use and questions to yourself. Continue expanding on your details, making notations in the margins regarding points you feel would benefit from audiovisual support. I use a small square to represent a slide or overhead. I then highlight the square so that it stands out visually. As the speech slowly makes the transition from bare outline to full presentation, I continue to use the highlighted square. When preparing your audiovisuals, this will remind you which points will need audiovisuals and how many audiovisuals you will use. During the presentation itself, these colored squares serve as a reminder to change the slide or overhead, so the point that I am making is the same one the audience is looking.

Now the speech must be converted to the format that will put you most at ease while you deliver your speech. How best to accomplish this varies from person to person. Although some speakers may feel comfortable utilizing note cards from which to speak, others feel it necessary to write out the entire speech first, and others still feel most comfortable working from a neatly typed outline. There are even a few speakers who will memorize what they have to say. Recognition of one's own personal style will direct a speaker down the proper path. There are advantages as well as disadvantages to each format.

Writing out the entire speech helps "crystallize your ideas, organize your thoughts, and identify gaps in logic and substance."[10] In addition, it is also useful if you are called on to deliver the same speech a few months down the line or to convert your presentation to a publication. On the other hand, reading a prepared speech "robs a presentation of spontaneity,"[16] as well as sounding

stilted.[2,17] If you opt to use a written text when you speak, the pages should be loose leaf, rather than stapled or clipped. Turning papers that are clipped together can be quite distracting and noisy. Some speakers utilize small three-ring binders to hold the pages. In addition, the pages should be numbered at the top, so that if they are accidentally dropped, you can easily reassemble them.

A neatly typed outline works wonderfully for well-rehearsed speakers who are very comfortable with their topic. The speaker need only glance at the outline to keep on track and can recite the details because of their familiarity with the topic. However, when the topic is highly sensitive or controversial so that exact phraseology is important, an outline can fail to offer enough support to a speaker. In addition, the speaker must be very well versed on the topic and relaxed enough that the relative lack of notes is not perturbing.

Note cards work well for many speakers. Note cards should include the outline, as well as key words, concepts, and phrases to guide you. Some speechwriters first write out their entire speech and then paraphrase it onto the cards. Limit the amount of information on each note card because they become more difficult to read with an increasing density of words; at that point, they have essentially become the text of your speech written out on cards. Note cards work best when typed or, at minimum, legibly hand lettered,[16] because this will increase your ability to pick out the key words and phrases at a glance. Note cards should also be numbered at the top for the same reasons as a written text. Although note cards are sufficient for many speakers, the novice speaker may not feel comfortable with this "Reader's Digest" version of their speech to support them.

Memorization of a speech is rarely recommended. A memorized speech makes the audience feel disconnected[10] from the speaker. In addition, if you lose your place, most people will need to go back to the beginning of the speech to proceed, which clearly most audiences would not appreciate.

Regardless of which style you are most comfortable with, it is crucial to recognize that spoken English and written English are quite different animals. For this reason, there are those speech-makers who do not write out the entire text of their speech, for fear of having it sound like a manuscript reading. At any rate, you would be well advised as you prepare your speech to write the way you speak; don't speak the way you write! Use plain English, use the familiar word or phrase rather than the fancy one, and use short words rather than long words.[18]

Preparation of Audiovisuals

Because most of us are visual learners, visual aids can be of great benefit to a speaker. Seventy-five percent of what we know is delivered visually, 13% audibly, and 12% through smell, taste, and touch.[10] There is an old Japanese proverb that speaks to this: "One seeing is better than a hundred times telling about."[9]

This is not to say, however, that audiovisuals must always be used. For instance, when delivering a keynote speech, many speakers purposely do not use audiovisuals. They want the audience to concentrate 100% on what they are saying. Many of these speakers will use, however, a background projected onto a screen behind them. For those presenting in a very large room, sometimes it is a projection of the speaker themselves as captured by a live-action camera. This enables the entire audience to capture facial gestures and mannerisms, allowing them to receive the full impact of the speaker's message. One researcher[19] who developed a formula to account for the emotional impact of any speaker calculated that the spoken word contributes 7% to emotional impact, vocal elements (pitch, speed, volume, etc.) 38%, and facial expressions 55%.

Other keynote speakers use a projection of the name of the organization, conference, or the title of the speech. Still others choose to use a single visual image of a symbolic object (e.g., a speech on peace backlit by an image of a dove with an olive branch). One of the golden rules of visual aids is to only use them if you need them; don't use them just to have them.[20,21]

Audiovisuals should always supplement your presentation, never substitute for it. Remember, it is you using the audiovisuals, and not vice versa. As one speaker put it, "It is always annoying when

the media is far more impressive than the speaker. In this case, send the media only and you stay home."[22] You should also never rely entirely on the audiovisuals to advance the presentation nor to clarify a point. If technology fails, your speech should be able to continue regardless.

As mentioned previously, the type of audiovisuals you use will be dictated by those details you wish to highlight, as well as the size of both the audience and the room. The most commonly used audiovisuals are printed handouts, overhead projections, slides, and Microsoft PowerPoint® LCD presentations. Other aids less commonly used include chalkboards, flip charts, and props, such as a model airway or a wrecked bicycle. Before investing hours creating your masterpiece, check with the sponsoring organization to make sure that the appropriate equipment will be available. It is always a disconcerting feeling to have prepared the finest audiovisuals, only to arrive and find yourself with top-notch slides and no projector.

Handouts are best utilized with smaller audiences and when there are many technical details to recall. Audiences do tend to like handouts because it provides them with something to take back to work to share, as well as being an easy reference. Handouts should always include your bibliography or reference list. Avoid distributing handouts to a large audience because the rustle of turning pages can be quite distracting. If there is a reference list you feel would be beneficial to issue when speaking to a large audience, have it available for distribution following the presentation.

Overheads are best used for small, informal group presentations. One advantage of using overheads is the ability to keep the room lighter than is possible with slides. This helps the speaker maintain eye contact, as well as discouraging napping! Another advantage is that overhead projectors are readily available, and there are few working parts to fail. If you use overheads, always mount them on frames, which makes them easier to move.[20] In addition, overheads should be numbered. This aids the speaker should they fall, as well as providing an easy way to reference them in the text of the speech. Additionally, know how to obtain an extra bulb for the overhead projector, should the bulb have less stamina than do you. Do not

use overheads if you have an audience of more than 50 people because the resolution is not strong enough for that large a group.

Color slides are an excellent method of holding an audience's attention. They tend to be expensive to produce, however, and for a one-time speech, producing them may exceed your cost-benefit ratio. Also, if you are asked to give the same speech in the future and any of the information has changed, you will need to get new slides made, which again can be rather costly. Another downside is that there are more "pieces" to fail. If you are using slides, make sure there is an extra projector bulb available. You should also make sure that the sponsors have the projector positioned properly, close enough to a power outlet to avoid making the cord a tripping hazard, or use an extension cord. Ideally, slides should be advanced with a remote control device, thus avoiding the cord hazard; many lecterns in large auditoriums have these projector controls built in. You should also always have a corded control available as well. When all else fails, you can use the button on the projector to advance the slides. If you are not located near the projector, try to find someone you know in the audience or a member of the sponsoring organization to perform this function.

Computerized presentations such as Microsoft PowerPoint® are becoming increasingly popular. These presentations are excellent at keeping an audience's attention because words fly in and pictures fade out. One key advantage of these presentations is that they are very easy to update, with no associated cost to do so, so your presentation never becomes outdated. Another advantage is the ability of some software programs to insert a video clip directly into a "slide." This can be a very powerful graphic representation of a clinical procedure. One shortcoming is that this adds one more piece of technology that can fail. Although the projectors necessary for these presentations are becoming more commonplace, they are still quite expensive and may not always be available.

Regardless of which type of audiovisual you opt for, they should vary in content between text visuals and picture visuals to help keep audience attention. In addition, the amount of information on each audiovisual should be limited. Crowded vi-

sual aids can detract from the speaker's message if there is so much information on the screen that the audience is busy reading what is displayed, rather than listening to what is said.

In addition, there are other key principles for maximizing effectiveness of the audiovisual presentation. Make sure that everyone in the audience can see the audiovisuals. Use words and phrases rather than full sentences to avoid the reading phenomenon. Use color and pictures to help hold audience interest. Use a larger font, as well as one that is sufficiently plain so that the words are easily readable. Avoid using all capitals because this is harder to read than a mix of upper- and lowercase letters.

There are additional rules for the speaker utilizing slides. Utilize the 5 x 7 x 7 rule: no more than 5 words in the title, no more than 7 words in width, and no more than 7 lines in height.[10] Also, research demonstrates that slides are most readable when the background is dark and the lettering is light; for this reason, a yellow font on a dark blue background will be easier for the audience to read than black letters on a white background.

The most powerful visual aids present congruent auditory and visual messages.[10] The visual aid must display only the point you are currently discussing; therefore, display only that visual aid. When you move on to the next point, either move on to the next visual aid or turn the machine off to avoid having the audience hear one message and see another. If you have five points to discuss, use five overheads or five slides. An additional option exists for those utilizing Microsoft Power-Point® technology. As you move to each point, have the previous point fade out or have the current point move forward. Perfecting these aspects of a computer-enhanced presentation can add punch to your delivery and help make your presentation more memorable.

Having completed the audiovisuals you intend to use, you must now go back to your speech and make sure you know where to display them. First, I put my audiovisuals in the order that they appear in the speech. Next, I go slowly through my speech to find the exact point at which I want that audiovisual to appear. Remember, we want

to avoid splitting the audience's attention, so we want to avoid putting up a slide or overhead before we are ready to talk about it. When I reach the point in the speech at which I should advance to the first slide, I make a small highlighted "box" in the margin. When I am using overheads, I go one step further. I number the overheads, again in the order in which they will be used. I then place the number of the overhead in the highlighted box. This enables me, at any point within the speech, to know what slide or overhead should be on the screen. If at one point you want the screen to go dark, indicate this in the margin as well.

Other helpful notes to write in the margins have to do with gestures or stage movements. If you remember back to the last play in which you participated, you will remember that the script directed you upstage, stage left, and so forth. If you want to ensure that you are moving about or that there is a specific gesture that you want to use to reinforce a point, write it in the margin. I then highlight this, using a different color than the audiovisual highlights.

The last notes I put in the margins have to do with timing. If I know my speech should last 1 hour, I put a small clock in the margin, with the hands highlighted at 15 minutes, 30 minutes, and so on. After practicing the speech many, many times, I know at what point I need to be at the 15-minute mark to finish the speech in one hour. Of course, I use yet another color for the clocks, so I know as I glance at my notes while speaking that yellow highlighting alerts me to change the slide or overhead, green means I should remember to walk away from the lectern, and pink means I should do a time check.

Personal Preparation

Once your speech is prepared and your audiovisuals created, it is time to prepare the most important ingredient, you! Even the most experienced speakers practice their speeches. This practice should occur in a stepwise manner. The first step consists of reading the speech out loud to yourself. Do the words sound as you thought they would, or do they sound stilted? Perhaps the opening joke is funny on paper, but lacks some-

thing on presentation. This is one more opportunity to fine-tune your presentation. The other purpose of practicing out loud is to become so familiar with the speech that it flows as easily off your tongue as an introduction of your immediate family members.

Once you are fairly certain that the speech says what you want it to say, and you are comfortable with all of the pronunciations and timing, it is time to practice in front of some good friends. These should be friends who are close enough to not tease you about mistakes, yet feel comfortable enough to offer suggestions for improving your presentation. Practice in front of several different groups of friends, and gather their suggestions on both content and presentation. I have found that, as the writer, a phrase makes perfectly obvious sense to me, but absolutely no sense at all to anyone else. This is yet another opportunity to fine-tune your address.

A great next step is to audiotape your speech. Tape recorders are inexpensive and are readily available. Taping your speech, just as you intend to deliver it, allows you to take the audience's seat to listen to you. Listen for timing. Are you rushing your delivery or pausing for effect at intervals? How many times did you say "uhm" or "ah"? How is your pronunciation? Mispronunciation of words detracts from a speaker's credibility; therefore, make sure that you look up the pronunciation of any words about which you are unsure.

Other things to listen for are pitch, pace, and volume. Your voice will always sound more nasal to you than to the audience,[23] so be prepared for this. The voice you hear on the audiotape may also sound higher in pitch than you expect. When stressed, people tend to talk faster and in a higher pitch. Therefore, you may need to concentrate on lowering your pitch, as well as slowing down your pace. Because of the adrenaline rush most speakers experience the day of the speech, you may very well deliver the speech faster than you do during practice or vice versa. You should try to determine your "practice speech to real speech" time ratio.[10] This will help you determine where to realistically place your time markers in your speech notes, as well as to make adjustments on the amount of content that you prepare.

You should also listen to determine if your pace is even or if it goes in spurts. Volume is also clearly an important factor. You should be loud enough to be heard, but not so loud that you sound as if you are shouting your speech from the mountaintop. If you know you tend to be soft spoken, make sure there will be a microphone available to help augment your volume.

Lastly, if you have the ability to do so, videotape your presentation and then watch the video as if you were an audience member. If you are unable to videotape yourself, practice your presentation in front of a mirror. How is your eye contact? Ideally, you should be making eye contact with people across the entire room as you speak. Each person should feel as if they have been personally addressed. This, however, can strike fear into the hearts of many speakers. One alternative is to pick three points in the room, all located just above the audience's heads: one on the left side of the room, one at the back, and one on the right side of the room. As you speak, look at these predetermined points. The audience members will assume you are making eye contact with the person in the row behind them, and you won't have to look into the eyes of a stranger at one of the most anxiety-provoking moments of your life.

Due to anxiety, some speakers display various interesting tics or mannerisms when they speak. Watch for these on the video as well. It is important to remember that even experienced speakers can suffer from stage fright. They have learned, however, to look calm and confident when they speak. As one speaker describes, "They have learned to keep their butterflies in formation."[11] One way they accomplish this is by controlling their nervous gestures. Do not rock back and forth, play with the quarters in your pocket, or examine your manicure while speaking. As one style guru put it,[18] "A podium is an inappropriate place to complete your morning toilette, even though you only limit it to cleaning your ears. The area between your umbilicus and knees is off limits for your hands. Don't scratch." I recall being in the audience during a presentation by a class of first graders. They were all obviously nervous, but one girl especially so. Her mother had taken care to dress her in a pretty dress for the occasion, but the entire time she was on stage, she rocked back

and forth, lifting her skirt WAY up and down. Of course, I don't recall at all what she was saying, singing, or otherwise, but I can describe in detail her Powerpuff Girls® undergarments!

Watch the video for other visual faux pas. Watch for body language, posture, and note rustling. If you want the audience to have confidence in your expertise, you must portray that confidence. Speakers should stand up straight with shoulders back when presenting. "One should not," as the queen counsels her granddaughter in Disney's *The Princess Diaries*, "Shlump." Gesturing should come naturally and not be overexaggerated. Dress for the videotape as you plan to dress for the presentation. Watch for unintended clothing gaffes, such as buttons gapping or skirts riding up. Have you remembered to look around the room at your audience, or are you speaking to your audiovisuals? Although a podium, if present, is an ideal place to keep your lecture notes, it should not be used as a shield between you and the audience. You should ensure that you are not cemented behind the podium and walk easily across the stage while speaking. Walking and gesturing both help add emphasis to your message; in addition, walking helps ensure that the entire audience has a chance to see you clearly.

The final preparation you must make is your decision of what to wear. Remember that you only get once chance to make a first impression, and that impression begins before you embark on your lecture. One study analyzed the dynamics of verbal communication and found that 55% of interpersonal communication is directly related to how people look, such as facial expression and body language. Manner of speech, such as vocal quality, accounted for 38% and speech content for the remaining 7%.[23] Guidelines for clothing choice include choosing clothes that are professional, attractive on you, clean and well-pressed, and most importantly, in which you feel comfortable. Wearing something that makes you feel good helps you both feel and look confident.

Other things to consider when choosing attire are whether or not you will be videotaped, whether presenting indoors or outdoors, and the size of the room. If you will be videotaped, choose a color that contrasts with your skin. You may notice that you never see newscasters wearing white; they are trying to avoid looking washed out. If you will be outdoors, make sure your clothing is appropriate for the weather. It is hard to appear calm and confident when you are approaching either hypothermia or heatstroke. In addition, women should avoid wearing excessively high heels when presenting outside because the spikes may sink into the ground. Larger rooms require slightly more dramatic makeup, although we would still like to avoid the Bozo look. Keep jewelry to a minimum, and avoid bracelets, watches, or earrings that jingle like wind chimes. These can be distracting to the audience and cause them to focus more on your accouterments than on your message.

Presentation Day

To counteract Murphy's Law, prepare for every eventuality. If your presentation is on your laptop computer, back it up on a disc. If it is on a disk, make a second disk. Bring two copies of your lecture notes with you. If you are traveling to your speaking engagement by airplane, bring your computer, notes, and audiovisuals as carry-on luggage. For ladies, bring at least two pairs of stockings. In addition, you should bring a clock or a watch to place on the podium.

You should avoid having a large meal prior to speaking, but you should eat something. A blood sugar of 40 is not compatible with a coherent speech. Avoid caffeinated beverages as well as alcohol because both can cause the mouth to dry out.

To be completely comfortable and prepared, arrive early. This means that you must be absolutely certain that you know where you are going. Get detailed travel instructions prior to the day of the presentation; if you are really detail oriented, you may wish to drive it yourself prior to presentation day to get an exact travel time. If you think that one-half hour is long enough for your travel there, leave one and one-half hours ahead of time. You want to leave enough time for every travel mishap that has ever occurred and still arrive early enough to check out the room. Even better, if you are able to stay overnight at the site, you will avoid the aggravation of traffic jams.

Once you arrive, let the program sponsors know. Check each and every piece of equipment yourself. Ensure that it is not only functional, but also that you know how to work it. If you will be using a microphone, test it. Microphones should usually be about 6 inches away to avoid sibilance and feedback. If you are using a lapel mike, make sure you have something on which to fasten it, and that it will not impede your movement across the stage. Place the lectern where you want it now; once the audience assembles, you do not want to be mistaken for the stage crew. If your speech is longer than one-half hour or if you tend to have a particularly dry mouth, ask the program sponsor for a glass of water to keep at the podium. Pausing to take a sip of water is always acceptable.

If your presentation is to be taped, you should be asked to sign a waiver or release allowing the taping to proceed. If the presentation that you are giving is copyrighted, you may specify that you may not be videotaped. In addition, many people become so nervous when they know they are being taped that all of their preparations go to waste. Although this should be discussed well in advance of the speaking date, it is never too late to "Just say no."

Make sure that the lighting is the way you want it, and that the room will not be so dark that you can't see your way across the stage. To ensure that you stay on time, keep your watch or a small clock on top of the podium. Your times should correspond with the times in the margins your speech. Remember to glance at the clock every so often to see how you are doing in terms of time, though not so often that the audience feels as if you have another engagement to rush off to.

Because stress inhibits the secretion of antidiuretic hormone, take a last trip to the restroom about 15 to 20 minutes prior to your presentation. That is a good time as well to check your hair, your makeup, and your clothing. It is hard to convey confidence with the remains of a jelly doughnut on your jacket. The time is now at hand, and you must leave the relative safety of the restroom and make your final preparation for speaking. Take a few slow, deep breaths; remember that you have been asked to speak because you are the expert, and it is normal to be a little nervous. Your anxiety will decrease every time you make a presentation.

Postpresentation

Having successfully completed your presentation, thank the program coordinator for inviting you to speak, take a deep sigh of relief, and go home. Your work is not yet complete, however. To become more accomplished as a speaker, it is necessary to gather constructive suggestions and feedback on your presentation. Check with the program sponsor to make certain that they know where they should forward your speaker evaluations. If friends or colleagues were in attendance, actively seek their feedback on both content and style. Keep a list of all of the feedback that you receive. This will be an effective tool when you prepare your next presentation.

Although the fear of public speaking prevents many intelligent and accomplished APNs from conducting formal presentations, by following an organized approach, such as outlined here, any nurse can achieve an impressive, successful, minimal-stress lecture.

REFERENCES

1. Knowles, E. (Ed.). (1999). *The Oxford dictionary of quotations*. Oxford, England: Oxford University Press.
2. Elsea, J. G. (1989). Communicate skillfully, successfully, and confidently. A ten-step process. *Clinical Laboratory Management Review, 3*(4), 201–205.
3. Laidlaw, M. (1993). Public speaking: A tool for career advancement. *Leadership in Health Services, 2*(4), 33–34.
4. Johnson, J. R. (1994). The communication training needs of registered nurses. *The Journal of Continuing Education in Nursing, 25*(5), 213–218.
5. Honeycutt, J., & Worobey, J. (1987). Impressions about communication styles and competence and nursing relationships. *Communication Education, 36*, 217–227.
6. Frone, M., & Major, B. (1988). Communication quality and job satisfaction among managerial nurses: The moderating influence of job involvement. *Group and Organizational Studies, 13*, 332–347.
7. Pincus, J. D. (1986). Communication satisfaction, job satisfaction, and job performance. *Human Communication Research, 12*, 395–419.
8. Kazemek, E. A., & Dauner, J. F. (1987). Overcoming the fear of public speaking. *Healthcare Financial Management, 41*(7), 104, 109.
9. Davis, J. H. (1998). Public speaking for fun and profit. *Journal of Emergency Nursing, 24*(1), 81–82.
10. Winslow, E. H. (1993). 20 tips to improve public speaking. *Orthopaedic Nursing, 12*(2), 15–18.
11. Wolf, Z. R., & Donnelly, G. F. (1993). Public speaking: Content and process evaluation of nursing students' presentations. *Nurse Educator, 18*(2), 30–32.

12. Fondiller, S. (1994). Public speaking: Try it—you'll like it. *American Journal of Nursing, 94*(3), 64–67.

13. Tuson, G. (1991). The art of public speaking. *Health Estate Journal, 45*(3), 12–18.

14. Michel, E., & Henley, J. (1989). Facing down the fear of public speaking. *RN, 52*(4), 19–21.

15. Smith, M. F. (2000). Public speaking survival strategies. *Journal of Emergency Nursing, 26*(2), 166–168.

16. McConnell, C. R. (2000). Speak up: The manager's guide to oral presentations. *Health Care Manager, 18*(3), 70–77.

17. Kelsey, B. (1984). Public speaking: Mastering the spotlight. *Association Management, 36*(4), 87–89.

18. Lambrecht, L. G., & Kalivoda, F. J. (1981). Public speaking: Replace insecurity with persuasiveness. *Radiology Management, 4*(1), 10–12.

19. Pagana, K. D., & Gingrow, K. S. (1990). A practical plan for teaching oral communication skills. *Nurse Educator, 15*(1), 17–19.

20. Madden, D. L. (1991). Public speaking: A fate worse than death? *The Internist, 32*(8), 30–31.

21. Howe, J. (1994). The Standard guide to public speaking. *Nursing Standard, 8*(44), 44–45.

22. Nelson, M., & Nelson, S. (1999). What? Me speak in public: What if somebody sees me? *Hospital Materiel Management Quarterly, 20*(4), 90–98.

23. Buxman, K., & Lemons, C. (1991). Fighting the fear of public speaking. *Nursing, 21*(8), 108, 110, 112.